Feeding Baby

Newborn to 24 Months

Including breast feeding, baby formula, store bought vs. homemade baby food, recipes, equipment, kitchenware, natural food, organic food, charts, scheduling, and much more!

By: Cynthia Cherry

Copyrights and Trademarks

All rights reserved. No part of this book may be reproduced or transformed in any form or by any means, graphic, electronic, or mechanical, including photocopying, recording, taping, or by any information storage retrieval system, without the written permission of the author.

This publication is Copyright © 2013. All products, graphics, publications, software and services mentioned and recommended in this publication are protected by trademarks. In such instance, all trademarks & copyright belong to the respective owners.

Disclaimer and Legal Notice

This product is not legal, medical, or accounting advice and should not be interpreted in that manner. You need to do your own due-diligence to determine if the content of this product is right for you. While every attempt has been made to verify the information shared in this publication, neither the author, neither publisher, nor the affiliates assume any responsibility for errors, omissions or contrary interpretation of the subject matter herein. Any perceived slights to any specific person(s) or organization(s) are purely unintentional.

We have no control over the nature, content and availability of the web sites listed in this book. The inclusion of any web site links does not necessarily imply a recommendation or endorse the views expressed within them. We take no responsibility for, and will not be liable for, the websites being temporarily unavailable or being removed from the internet.

The accuracy and completeness of information provided herein and opinions stated herein are not guaranteed or warranted to produce any particular results, and the advice and strategies, contained herein may not be suitable for every individual. Neither the author nor the publisher shall be liable for any loss incurred as a consequence of the use and application, directly or indirectly, of any information presented in this work. This publication is designed to provide information in regard to the subject matter covered.

Neither the author nor the publisher assume any responsibility for any errors or omissions, nor do they represent or warrant that the ideas, information, actions, plans, suggestions contained in this book is in all cases accurate. It is the reader's responsibility to find advice before putting anything written in this book into practice. The information in this book is not intended to serve as legal, medical, or accounting advice.

Forward

As a new parent you will experience a moment that is both wonderful and terrifying. It is that instant of realization that for your baby, you are "it." This tiny, wonderful little person you haven't even yet come to know is looking to you to fulfil its every need — safety, warmth, love, and food.

Your own body will not yet have recovered from the experience of pregnancy. Your hormones are all over the place. Even if you are not suffering from postpartum depression you will experience a cascade of emotions in the beginning, some that may even make you doubt your fitness as a mother.

Although he has not gone through the physical experience of carrying the baby, your husband or partner is likely feeling the same kind of roller coaster of elation and doubt.

All new parents experience this confusing transition, but mothers in particular have a tendency to put more on themselves than they can really handle. This is especially true when the child is your first.

Our society is very good at creating false images of "perfection." The media bombards us with stories of apparently flawless celebrities "doing" parenthood better than it's ever been done before. All too often, that leaves the rest of us feeling inadequate and more than a little second rate.

Forward

Every mother wants to make sure that their child receives positively golden care. The desire is for everything the child sees, hears, smells, and tastes to be nothing but the purest and the best.

New mothers have a tendency — before the exhaustion kicks in — to convince themselves that they can tackle childrearing better than it's ever been done before.

One of my goals in writing this book is to help new mothers set realistic goals. Your number one priority is nurturing your child, but you mustn't lose sight of your own needs.

As much as we women hate to admit it, there is no such thing as perfection. As the mother of three children, I can assure you it's okay to give yourself a break. "Disasters" tend to occur much more often when you don't!

We also have to accept that children are being raised in a very changed world. Food isn't really food anymore, so it's no longer just an issue of deciding to breast feed or not to breast feed.

I wasn't breast fed as a child. I did try to breast feed my first child, but was unable to produce enough milk to keep up with my baby's needs. So, I switched to formula and exclusively used formula for my other two children as well.

At the time of my first pregnancy, a number of well-meaning souls presumed to judge me for my choice, but I got over what I perceived to be hurtful comments with

Forward

close family support. I have no doubt that my experience is not unique.

If I were raising a baby today, I suspect the criticisms would come just as readily on subjects like additives, chemicals, and genetically modified organisms.

It's hard to feed ourselves in a healthy way, so understand that this text will proceed without judgment. The only real goal is good, solid nutrition for your baby that creates the optimum climate for a life of excellent health.

With that in mind, I have included a section on alternate feeding approaches, including going vegan. The "right" choice is the one that works for you, your spouse, and your child.

If I were to ask you to move into the main body of the text with one thought in mind, it would be this. Every pregnancy is different. Every baby is different and every mother is different.

My purpose in writing this book is to give you the information you need to make your own choices and your own decisions without stress and guilt.

(Please note that from time to time the text uses male pronouns to refer to babies. This is simply a reflection of the fact that I took high school English when the universal male reference was still the accepted standard. I certainly don't mean to neglect the girls or to be politically incorrect. It's just an old habit!)

Acknowledgments

I would like to express my gratitude towards my family, friends, and colleagues for their kind co-operation and encouragement which helped me in completion of this book.

I would like to express my special gratitude and thanks to my loving husband for his patience, understanding, and support.

My thanks and appreciations also go to my colleagues and people who have willingly helped me out with their abilities.

Additional thanks to my children, whose love and my concern for their wellbeing inspired me to write this book.

Table of Contents

Forward 1

Acknowledgments 5

Table of Contents.. 7

Part I: Age 0-6 Months, Breast Milk or Formula 11

    Deciding to Breastfeed... 12

    Considering the Middle Ground 13

    Myths and Misconceptions About Breastfeeding 14

    Breast Feeding is a Choice 16

    How-To: Breastfeeding Basics....................................... 17

    How-To: Store Breast Milk 20

    Selecting Nursing Pads 22

    Buying Nursing Bras 23

    Buying Breast Pumps 24

    When to Stop Breastfeeding 26

    Formula Isn't "Second Rate" Nutrition 27

    Putting Formula in Perspective..................................... 28

    Whole Cow's Milk.. 29

    Modern Baby Formula 31

    Selecting a Baby Formula.. 32

    Ignore Advertising Hype 33

    What Not to Ignore 33

Table of Contents

Four Major Types of Formula 34
    Cow's Milk 34
    Soy Based 35
    Protein Hydrolysate 35
    Specialty Formulas 35

Formula Product Formats 36
    Powdered 36
    Concentrated Liquid 37
    Ready-to-Use 37

A Word on Water Supply 38

Buying Baby Bottles 42

How-To: Bottle Feeding Basics 45

Burping Your Baby 46

Part II – Age 6 Months - Introducing Solid Foods 49
    Vegetarian, Vegan and Gluten Free Cooking 54
    Watching for Food Allergies 55
    Where to Feed the Baby 56
    Considering Baby Food in Jars 57
    Deciding on Organic Foods 59
    Should You Buy Organic Produce? 60
    Storing Homemade Baby Food 64

Part III -Your Child's Nutritional Needs 69

Table of Contents

Simple and Complex Carbohydrates 70

Soluble and Insoluble Fiber 71

Complete and Incomplete Proteins 72

Saturated, Unsaturated, and Trans Fats 74

Vitamins and Minerals 76

Iron 78

Calcium 78

The Scoop on Poop 81

Part IV – 12 to 24 Months 85

Evolving Eating Skills 86

Scheduled Meals and Snacks 87

How Much Food? 87

Teething 89

Eating Practices 89

Recipes? Not Really 91

Afterword 95

Relevant Websites 99

Frequently Asked Questions 101

Glossary 109

Index 115

Table of Contents

Part I: Age 0-6 Months, Breast Milk or Formula

Expectant parents work hard at the pre-planning stage of having a baby. Some opt to know the gender of their child so they can buy all the right things and decorate accordingly.

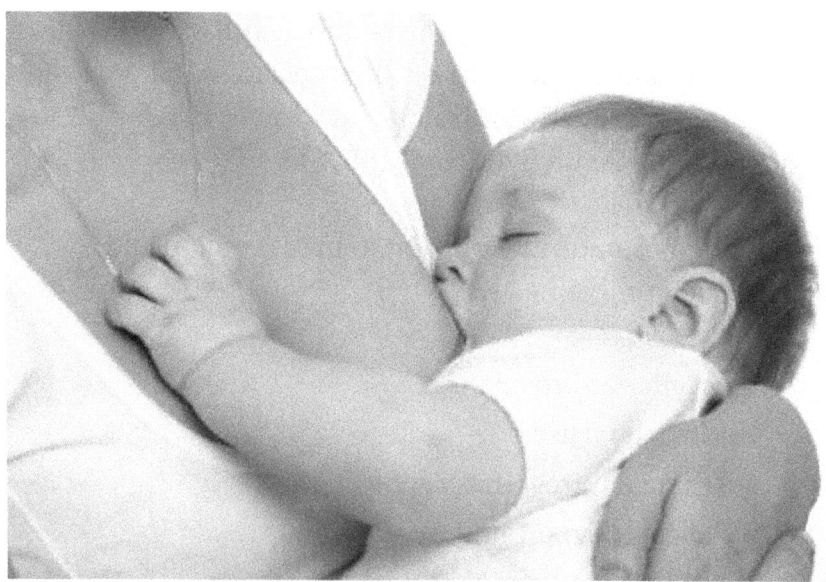

Amid all that preparation, most parents make carefully considered decisions about how they plan to feed their child — only to be brought up short when circumstances completely out of their control demand another approach.

It's perfectly fine to prepare to breastfeed (completely or in part) or to bottle feed, but allow yourself a window of opportunity to change your mind if you need to.

Part I: Age 0-6 Months, Breast Milk or Formula

If you haven't made the decision between feeding breast milk or formula to your baby, we need to discuss the major considerations for both nutritional approaches.

Deciding to Breastfeed

There are many well-documented reasons to opt to breastfeed your child. A mother's milk is full of antibodies that will help her child fight off diseases. Researchers even believe that breastfed children are at a lower risk for Sudden Infant Death Syndrome (SIDS).

The antibodies naturally present in breast milk protect against such problems as:

- chronic ear infections
- stomach viruses
- asthma and respiratory infections
- diabetes (Type 1 and 2)
- childhood leukemia

Studies also indicate that breastfed children are at a lower risk for the development of obesity over their lifetime.

Interestingly, the benefits are felt by the mother as well. Mothers who breast feed show a decreased risk for developing breast and ovarian cancers, struggle less with postpartum depression, and gain protection against diabetes.

Part I: Age 0-6 Months, Breast Milk or Formula

Typically, babies digest breast milk more easily. Some commercial formulas are made from cow's milk (albeit low fat cow's milk), which contains proteins infants may have difficulty tolerating at first.

That being said, there are a number of advantages to formula feeding:

- The ability to monitor exactly how much the child is eating.

- Shielding the infant from side effects from any foods the mother is eating, illnesses she experiences, or medications she requires.

- Allowing all members of the family to participate in feedings, facilitating more bonding time with both parents and siblings.

Since babies eat slightly less often when fed formula, the number of feedings per day decreases somewhat, which may better match some family's schedules.

Considering the Middle Ground

Some people fail to realize that there is a middle ground position, partial breastfeeding. This is not an all or nothing proposition.

Partial breastfeeding works especially well for mothers who are having difficulty producing enough milk and for

Part I: Age 0-6 Months, Breast Milk or Formula

working mothers who simply cannot find the time they need to breastfeed or to express milk.

There is no set rule for deciding how much breast milk your child receives opposed to the baby's intake of formula. Advocates of breastfeeding are universal in saying some breast milk is always better than none.

If you are considering partial breast feeding, mitigating factors to consider might include such things as:

- the working schedule of one or both parents
- how much breast milk can be successfully expressed and stored on a regular basis
- the quantity of milk you are actually able to produce

It is generally recommended, however, that if at all possible the child receive four weeks of exclusive breastfeeding before any formula is introduced.

Myths and Misconceptions About Breastfeeding

Often our beliefs about any topic, especially one as emotionally charged as breastfeeding, are deeply influenced by the opinions that are dominant in our culture — even if those ideas are actually *myths*.

Inadequate Milk Production?

The idea that many women cannot produce enough milk is certainly a misconception. Actually, the exact opposite tends to be true.

Part I: Age 0-6 Months, Breast Milk or Formula

In cases where a child does not thrive on breastfeeding the real problem is almost always that the infant is poorly latched on. All mothers, but especially first time mothers, need instruction in helping their child breastfeed.

Women have been breastfeeding babies for centuries, but that doesn't mean that either the mother or the child know exactly what to do automatically.

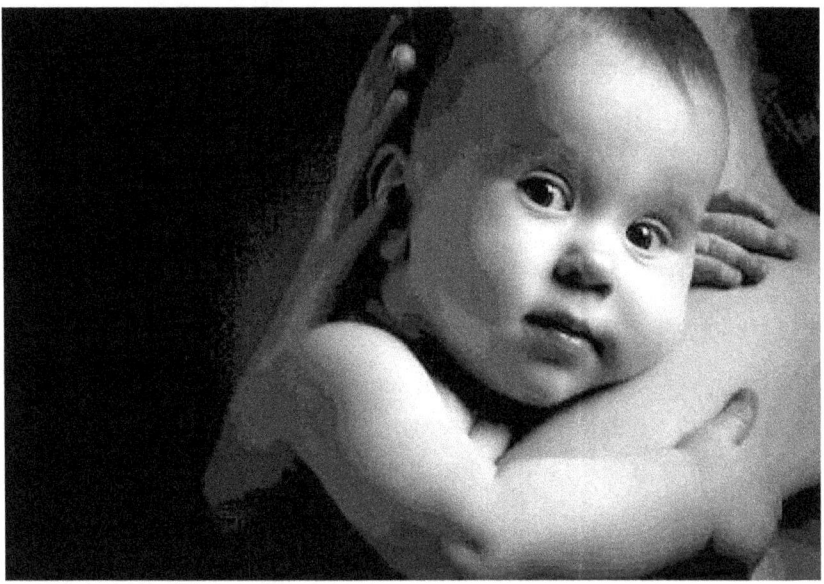

Lactation specialists and trainers can help enormously by simply observing a feeding and offering helpful instruction. This kind of training is typically available at the hospital where the child is delivered.

Modern Women Can't Produce Milk?

You will likely hear the absurd notion that modern women are no longer capable of nourishing their children

Part I: Age 0-6 Months, Breast Milk or Formula

exclusively from breast milk, or that an inability to produce adequate milk is an inherited trait. Neither of those "facts" is true either.

Humans are mammals. We are biologically designed to produce milk for our young. Problems with nursing can often be resolved by something as simple as nursing more frequently to stimulate production, offering both breasts during feeding, or massaging the breast gently while the child is suckling.

Breast Feeding is a Choice

In the midst of all this information, however, please don't lose sight of the fact that breastfeeding your baby is a choice. It has to work for you as well as for the child.

It's far too easy for a new mother to be shamed into breast feeding by doctors, nurses, family, and well-meaning friends. The truth is that some women just do not like to breast feed. That is perfectly fine.

There is no imperative to breast feed in order to qualify as a "perfect" mother. Your child will certainly know if you're uncomfortable or unhappy during feedings.

The optimal situation for you both is the one with the least amount of stress and the greatest amount of calm bonding time. If you are worried that formula will not meet your child's nutritional needs, there really is no need for that groundless fear to rule your decision.

Part I: Age 0-6 Months, Breast Milk or Formula

How-To: Breastfeeding Basics

Although many first-time mothers find it helpful to watch breast-feeding "how to" videos or to work with a lactation coach, these are the basics of positioning your child to latch on to the nipple for feeding.

Step One:

Find a comfortable location. Feeding times can vary significantly from 5-40 minutes. You want some place that is quiet with no distractions, especially in the beginning.

As you become more accustomed to feeding your child, you will be able to quietly read or listen to music through your headphones without upsetting your baby or disrupting the feeding time.

Step Two:

You can lie on your back to breast feed with your baby resting against your body, or cradle the child across your chest.

Have pillows or cushions ready if you are holding the child and your arm begins to tire. Make sure your back is well supported.

Step Three:

Bring the child to your breast with the head tipped back so that the baby is leading the motion with its chin. When the

Part I: Age 0-6 Months, Breast Milk or Formula

child's lips touch the nipple, the infant will instinctively drop the lower jaw. With a smooth, quick motion move the baby's mouth on to the breast.

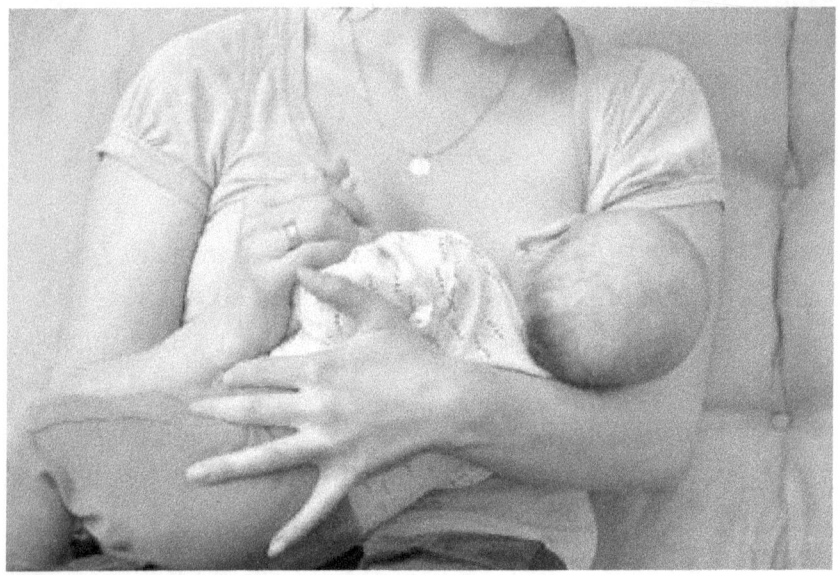

Pay attention to the sensation when your child takes the nipple. In latching on, the child should take a mouthful of tissue.

To ensure this is the case, the child's mouth should be wide open as it comes on the breast. Remember, the child's tongue, bottom lip, and chin makes initial contact. The bottom lip should be as far from the base of the nipple as possible.

If you experience pain, the baby is not latched on correctly. If this is the case, place your finger gently between your child's mouth and your breast to break the seal and begin again.

Part I: Age 0-6 Months, Breast Milk or Formula

Don't just carry on in a state of discomfort or your nipples will become too sore to properly feed your child.

You will know that the feeding is going well if the child progresses from short, quick sucks to slow, deep suckling. The child's head should be tipped back with the chin touching the breast with the nose free and clear.

There should be more of your areola visible above the child's upper lip than below the bottom one.

Step Four:

Allow your child to nurse for as long as the baby is hungry. The child should be relaxed and content, not wriggling around. The infant will release the breast when they are done.

Step Five:

At the end of the feeding examine your nipple. If it appears "squashed," it's likely it was not far enough back in the baby's mouth and you still need to improve the child's ability to latch on well.

The nipple should be at the back of the child's mouth where the hard palate ends. The child's jaw will move up and down with the action of the tongue to draw the milk into the mouth. The baby's lower gum should never touch the breast.

Part I: Age 0-6 Months, Breast Milk or Formula

Additional Tips:

Place your palm behind the child's shoulders and your index finger and thumb behind the ears to support the head and better direct the baby's motion toward the breast.

If the child's hands are in the way, try wrapping the infant in a blanket so the baby's arms are at the sides. This will let you keep the baby closer to the breast for more successful feedings.

Keep your hand away from your nipple as much as possible. Once the baby is properly supported and nursing, stay as still as you can.

When your child is sick, breastfeeding will supply needed comfort as well as nutrition and can help to settle a fussy baby.

How-To: Store Breast Milk

Before handling breast milk, always wash your hands thoroughly with soap and water. Breast milk should be stored in glass or hard plastic containers.

There are special bags designed for milk collection and storage that may also be a good option, however, bags are not ideal for long-term storage due to the potential for leaks and breakage.

Part I: Age 0-6 Months, Breast Milk or Formula

Be sure to label each container of milk with the date it was expressed. If the stored milk is to be taken to another site, be sure the label also includes your child's name.

Always store breast milk at the back of the refrigerator where the temperature will be at its coolest. Try to put just enough milk in each container for one feeding so there will be less waste.

A good starting point is 2-4 ounces (59-118 milliliters). You can adjust the amount as you become more familiar with your baby's feeding habits. It's always a good idea to store some smaller portions for irregular feedings.

It's alright to add additional milk to a portion that was expressed earlier in the day so long as the extra amount is allowed to cool completely.

Freshly expressed breast milk will keep at room temperature, (not to exceed 77°F / 25°C), for up to eight days in the refrigerator (at 32° - 39°F / 0° - 3.9°C) or in a cooler with ice packs for up to 24 hours. You can also freeze your breast milk for up to two weeks.

Make sure to leave a bit of room at the top of the bottle for expansion during freezing. Thaw your frozen milk by moving it to the refrigerator. It will take approximately 24 hours to thaw your milk.

If you plan to use the milk immediately, make sure to run warm water over the bag or bottle until it reaches room temperature. Never refreeze your breast milk.

Part I: Age 0-6 Months, Breast Milk or Formula

Selecting Nursing Pads

It's almost impossible for a breastfeeding mother to predict when or if she'll "leak." Having at least a package of nursing pads on hand is an excellent idea until you know more about how your body will function while producing milk.

Nursing pads can be purchased that are disposable or washable. You may actually want both. When you're away from home having disposable pads makes more sense, especially since you will always want a dry, clean pad on hand.

Airflow and absorbency are major considerations. Pick pads that are 100% cotton. Disposable pads should have multiple layers for maximum absorbency, but avoid plastic liners unless they are "breathable."

Don't use liquid fabric softener with reusable pads, or they won't take in as much liquid. Always remember that using a wet pad or one with poor airflow increases the risk of yeast infections. Always discard wet pads and put fresh ones in place as soon as possible.

Bigger pads are more discreet under clothing, and pads that are pink will be less visible. Disposable pads have the advantage of adhesive backings to help them stay securely in place.

Part I: Age 0-6 Months, Breast Milk or Formula

Buying Nursing Bras

Women are used to the idea that their regular clothes won't fit as their pregnancy progresses, but many aren't prepared for requiring new lingerie. By at least the 16th week of the pregnancy, your bra will no longer be sufficient to support your breasts.

By the second trimester, you will likely need to be fitted for new bras yet again, and by the final weeks of your pregnancy you'll want to have your nursing bras purchased.

Shopping at a maternity shop is the best way to get the right advice on fit and materials. These stores have fitters trained in helping pregnant women. Just increasing the size of your regular fashion bra will not work and will likely increase your level of discomfort.

The cups of a nursing bra provide access to the breast for your baby. You want to make sure that you can open the flap one-handed, so pay particular attention to the type of closure. Select bras that are 100% cotton or a breathable cotton or Lycra blend.

While it may be tempting to scrimp on the cost of your nursing bra based on the reasoning that you won't be using it for long, don't give in to that type of thinking. Get a good, quality bra that won't place pressure on your milk ducts increasing the chance of a blockage.

Part I: Age 0-6 Months, Breast Milk or Formula

For this reason, lactation specialists are against nursing bras with underwires. If you are used to an underwire, find a nursing bra with a flexible plastic underwire, but have another bra on hand without the wire insert in case the wire does prove to be uncomfortable over time.

Buying Breast Pumps

Breast pumps are typically recommended in the beginning to increase milk production. A pump can be an excellent tool, but it isn't always necessary.

Many women do choose to pump even when their child is feeding well simply to reinforce the "message" to their breasts. The best strategy, however, is the one that fits your goals.

You can use a pump for a few weeks to maximize production, or to have breast milk on hand for your child when you can't be present for feedings.

Choosing a pump can be a difficult decision, especially for new mothers. Hospital grade pumps, although too expensive to purchase at $700-$1500 / £432 - £925 are the most efficient.

These units can be rented for $40-$80 / £25 - £50 a month and are used with personal attachment kits that are purchased separately. The major manufacturers of this class of device are Ameda and Medela.

Part I: Age 0-6 Months, Breast Milk or Formula

Consumer grade electric pumps are single user and come in a variety of capacities. On the higher end, these units have dual pumping settings at full suction, and can be highly effective. These units are priced in the $150-$350 / £93 - £216 range.

A good pump is one with a strong mix of suction, strength, and cycling speed. If a pump reaches full pressure too quickly, for instance, it can cause tissue damage, but so can a unit that builds its suction too slowly.

Overall, experts agree that renting a hospital grade pump is the best option. The smaller, less expensive pumps wear out or break down, and they don't draw milk out efficiently.

In many cases, an older manual pump can be more effective than a brand new, but low-quality electric pump. Since the rule is always to get the best tool you can afford, the best in this case is a rented hospital grade pump.

You will likely have to experiment with multiple flange sizes as friction will cause soreness, as will allowing the pump to take in too much tissue. The majority of women do well with a 27-29 mm flange.

It is even possible to use the oldest method of extracting milk, hand expression, which is an art that comes quite naturally to some women. If this traditional methods works for you, it should be performed with the same frequency and duration as with a mechanical pump.

Part I: Age 0-6 Months, Breast Milk or Formula

Regardless, you should pump both breasts simultaneously to get the greatest volume. Nurse your child for as long as the baby will eat, and then pump.

When to Stop Breastfeeding

There are no set rules about when to stop breastfeeding. Mothers who make the decision to continue offering their child breast milk into the second year of life may have to deal with social criticism, but the truth is that medical science does come down in their favor.

Breastfeeding lowers the risk of many childhood diseases, and also mitigates the long-term risks of cardiovascular disease, diabetes, and degenerative disorders of the nervous system like multiple sclerosis.

Breast fed children are more slender, have better vision, experience fewer ear infections, and have stronger dental health. They have better digestion with less vomiting, acid reflux, and constipation and have a stronger immune system.

A child's brain triples in size from birth to age two. Breast milk contains omega-3 fatty acids, in particular DHA, which enhances brain development.

The World Health Organization actually recommends that mothers feed their children up to age three! So, bottom line, if it's working for you and your child, breastfeed until YOU think it's time to stop.

Part I: Age 0-6 Months, Breast Milk or Formula

Formula Isn't "Second Rate" Nutrition

While breast milk is optimal, modern day baby formulas are not second rate nutrition. These products are themselves based on the nutrient values and levels found in breast milk.

Over the last two decades there has been tremendous pressure placed on women to breast feed, but studies conducted in 2012 found that setting achievable goals is much more realistic and beneficial -- even if only partial breast feeding is possible.

In part, the high nutritional quality of currently available baby formula influenced the outcome of these findings. "Judgments" of both formula and breast milk are far more relative than once believed.

Researchers are now more directly confronting the fact that breast milk itself is far from "standard" in composition and can even vary in "quality" from one feeding to the next.

For instance, the amount of fat in breast milk is affected by the mother's daily intake. Any nutritional deficiency present in the mother will be reflected in her milk.

A baby's changing nutritional requirements must also be considered. At four months, your child's need for iron increases sharply. Breast milk alone can no longer meet that requirement, nor will a mother's milk provide the necessary levels of Vitamin D.

Part I: Age 0-6 Months, Breast Milk or Formula

By six months, babies need greater amounts of protein. Regardless of the level of milk production of which the mother is capable, other food sources will need to be added to the child's diet at this time.

When you encounter recommendations for exclusive breastfeeding like those offered by the World Health Organization, it's important to remember that those goals are directed primarily toward mothers in underdeveloped nations with poor sanitation and hygienic.

In those environments, breast milk is crucial in improving a child's immune system and protecting against disease. These considerations do not necessarily apply in the developed world.

Putting Formula in Perspective

A hundred years ago when mothers could not nurse their babies, the services of a wet nurse were essential for the child's survival. Infant mortality rates were high because not everyone could afford to hire a nurse.

In the latter half of the 19th century this nutritional gap began to be addressed with baby formulas based on cow's milk. Justin von Liebig developed the first commercial formula in 1867, "Liebig's Soluble Food for Babies."

Over the next few years the recipes for these formulas included cow's milk, water, cream, sugar, and honey. The latter alone is cause for serious concern.

Part I: Age 0-6 Months, Breast Milk or Formula

Honey should never be given to children under one year of age because it contains the spores that cause botulism. The consequences of this exposure can be fatal to infants.

The emphasis in the recipes for these early formulas was based primarily on palatability. With high infant mortality rates in the absence of available wet nurses, the desire was to get children to eat – anything.

Apart from other real concerns, however, the fundamental problem with these first commercial formulas is the fact that they were based on cow's milk. Human babies should never be fed whole cow's milk.

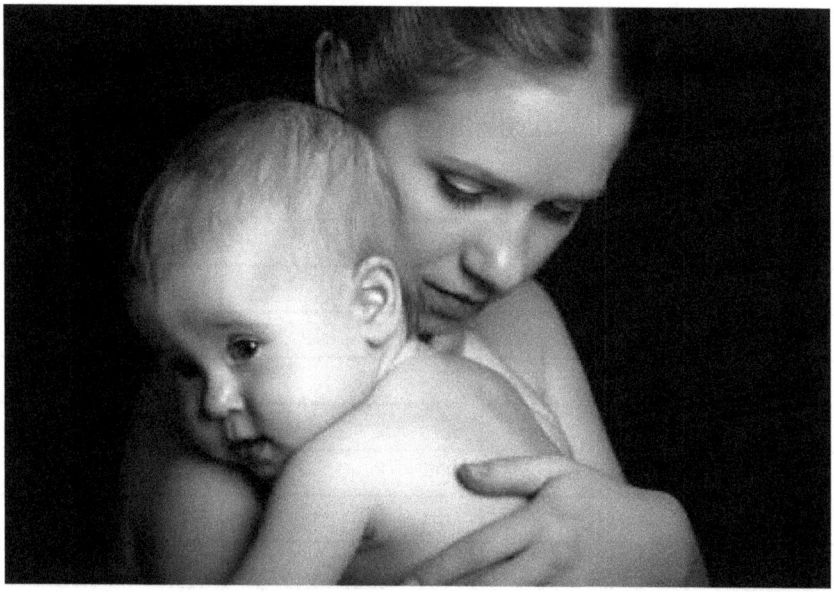

Whole Cow's Milk

Every species of mammal produces unique milk that is nutritionally tailored to the needs of that animal. A calf's

Part I: Age 0-6 Months, Breast Milk or Formula

needs and those of a human infant are decidedly not the same.

Simply consider the rate of development in the two "babies." Calves get up and start walking shortly after birth. Human babies come into the world at a much earlier and more vulnerable stage of growth.

Cow's milk contains levels of protein that are too high for human infants. Whole milk should never be given to a baby under 12 months of age due to a risk of intestinal blood loss that can lead to anemia.

Additionally, cow's milk contains 63% fatty acid content where breast milk has only 43%. Broken down in a comparison per 100 grams, this is how the two substances differ:

Nutritional Component	Cow's Milk	Human Milk
water	87.4	85.2
protein	3.5	1.1
calcium	118	33
phosphorous	93	14
sodium	50	16
potassium	144	51
Vitamin A	140	240
thiamine	0.03	0.01
riboflavin	0.17	0.04
niacin	0.1	0.2
ash	0.7	0.2

Feeding Baby

Part I: Age 0-6 Months, Breast Milk or Formula

There are numerous additional considerations with cow's milk:

- It forms large curds that digest slowly.

- The short chain fatty acids irritate the intestine.

- The high phosphorous content can cause convulsions.

- The level of ash leads to episodes of diarrhea.

- Qualitatively, cow's milk does not provide a good supply of iron. It has a low level of Vitamin A, and almost no Vitamin D unless it has been "fortified."

Vitamin A deficiency causes blindness in infants, while there is a link between insufficient Vitamin D and autism.

The National Academy of Sciences Institute of Medicine doubled the recommended levels for vitamin D intake in 2008, so even human breast milk will no longer meet this nutritional need.

Modern Baby Formula

As scientists began to understand and appreciate the developmental benefits of breast milk, they refined the accepted recipes for infant formula significantly.

Part I: Age 0-6 Months, Breast Milk or Formula

In the 1950s the first preparations using low-fat milk and vegetable oil were introduced, and more consideration was given to the quality of the proteins present in the milk used.

There are two categories of protein in milk, the casein faction and the whey faction. Casein is predominant in cow's milk at a level of 80%, while human breast milk is 60% whey and 40% casein.

Ultra-filtered whey proteins were first introduced into infant formulas in the 1970s, beginning a process of refinement that resulted in the highly sophisticated products available today.

Given this progressive development using human breast milk, not cow's milk as the nutritional gold standard, modern baby formulas will definitely give your child a good start in life even if no breast milk is available in the infant's diet.

Regardless of the amount of formula you decide to incorporate into your child's diet, you still have a huge hurdle before you – deciding which one to use!

Selecting a Baby Formula

While the whole breastfeeding vs. baby formula discussion may seem straightforward, when you walk into a store to purchase a baby formula, you may find yourself staring slack-jawed at the vast array of products.

Part I: Age 0-6 Months, Breast Milk or Formula

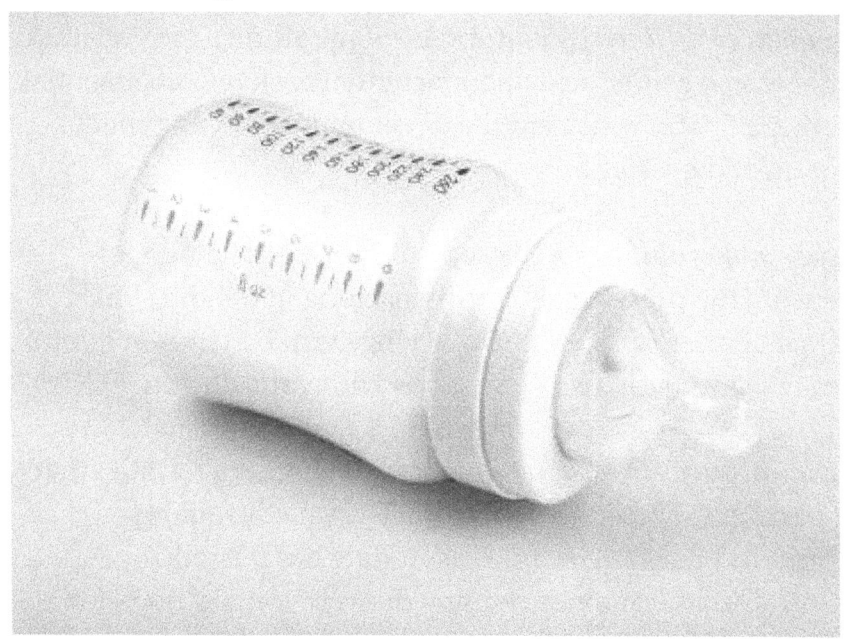

Ignore Advertising Hype

Over the past decade there has been a tremendous amount of public controversy over product labels on infant formulas. The manufacturing companies can and do make all sorts of claims about the added nutritional value of their products – most of which are completely unsubstantiated.

What Not to Ignore

The statements regarding formula content that you do not want to ignore include:

iron fortified – If you are not breastfeeding your child, an iron-fortified formula is necessary for the baby's growth and development.

Part I: Age 0-6 Months, Breast Milk or Formula

enhanced with DHA and ARA – Some studies indicate that docosahaxaenoic acid and arachidonic acide, both essential omega-3 fatty acids, aid the development of your child's brain and eyesight.

pre- and probiotics – These additives are intended to ensure the presence of healthy bacteria in the intestinal tract. Studies suggest positive long-term benefits, but you may want to discuss these foods with your doctor.

expiration date – Do not buy and never use a formula that is expired. There is no way to determine the quality of the product once the recommended date has passed. Examine all containers for any dents or bulges. Look for leaks and/or rust spots. Don't buy any formula in a container with these kinds of irregularities.

Four Major Types of Formula

There are four major types of baby formula currently available, which I will discuss below. Your first option will likely be a formula based on cow's milk.

If your child is not tolerant of this type of product, however, there are other choices of which you should be aware.

Cow's Milk

Formulas based on cow's milk have been modified to replicate human breast milk as nearly as possible, both for nutrient content and digestibility.

Part I: Age 0-6 Months, Breast Milk or Formula

These products should have the correct balance of protein, fat, and carbohydrates, and are designed to be as close to human breast milk as possible.

Soy Based

Soy-based formulas are an option for mothers who want their child's diet to be free of animal proteins. These preparations are also used in children that are allergic to or intolerant of cow's milk formulas.

Protein Hydrolysate

In protein hydrolysate formulas, the protein has been broken into smaller sizes than those present in cow's milk or soy products.

This enhances ease of digestion, making these formulas the "last resort" for children who have proven intolerant of cow's milk or soy-based formulas.

To further complicate the number of choices, formulas are available in three major form factors which I will discuss shortly.

Specialty Formulas

You will also see a plethora of "specialty" formulas, some for premature or "low birth weight" babies or those that are "metabolic" to deliver highly specialized nutrition.

Part I: Age 0-6 Months, Breast Milk or Formula

Do not select a specialty formula for your child without consulting with your pediatrician. These formulas should only be given to your child for a specific medical reason.

Make sure that you understand that reason, and have clear recommendations from your doctor on the correct specialty formula to feed your child, as well as the amount of and frequency of feedings.

Typically, when specialty formulas are indicated, you will be closely monitoring food intake and the child's weight and reporting these findings to your pediatrician.

The need for a specialty formula does not necessarily mean there is any serious health concern. Your baby may need more help to get over a case of colic, or to get relief from acid reflux.

Formula Product Formats

Infant formulas are available in three formats including powdered, concentrated liquids, and ready-to-use.

Powdered

Powdered infant formulas are the least expensive, but the most time consuming of all formulas. It is necessary to follow the preparation instructions exactly.

Many parents choose powdered formulas over concentrated liquids or ready-to-use varieties because the

Part I: Age 0-6 Months, Breast Milk or Formula

boxes do not contain bisphenol A (BPA), which is found in plastic containers and the lining of some cans.

In the body, BPA mimics estrogen and disrupts the endocrine system, which can harm brain and immune system development among other negative effects.

(Although powdered formulas circumvent the BPA worry, they do have to be mixed with water, which raises a whole new level of concern about toxicity. See the section below, "A Word on the Water Supply.")

Concentrated Liquid

Concentrated liquid formulas are mixed with water (generally in equal parts). In terms of expense, these are the middle ground products. They are slightly easier to use than powdered formula.

Ready-to-Use

Ready-to-use formulas are the most expensive option – about 20% more costly by volume – but they are also the most convenient.

Hospitals rely on ready-to-use formulas not only for ease of feeding, but also because the products, which require no mixing, are hygienic.

If you live in an area where the quality of the water supply is questionable, or if you are not comfortable with the

Part I: Age 0-6 Months, Breast Milk or Formula

available water supply, ready-to-use formulas are your best option.

Note that once opened, a ready-to-use formula must be given to the child within 48 hours or discarded.

A Word on Water Supply

Since some infant formulas have to be mixed or diluted with water – and since your growing child needs water – you must seriously consider the fact that "plain" water may be one of the most dangerous things your child can encounter.

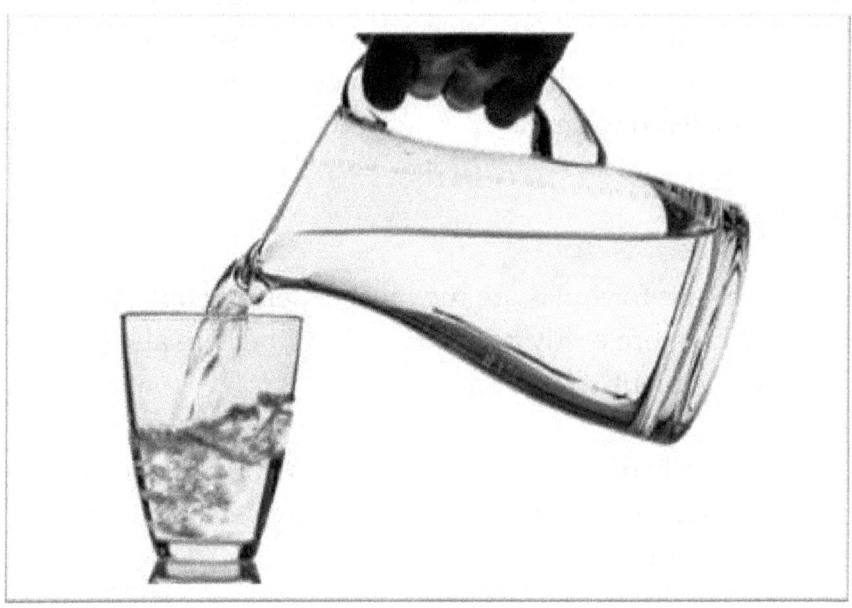

In August 2013, the Environmental Working Group released a report, "Water Treatment Contaminants: Toxic

Part I: Age 0-6 Months, Breast Milk or Formula

Trash in Drinking Water," based on an analysis of samples taken from municipal water systems in 43 states in the United States.

Every one of the systems tested positive for chemicals the report labelled "probably human carcinogens." The problem, however, is more sinister and extensive.

Chlorine, and other chemicals used to "treat" water to make it safe for human consumption interact with organic particles in the water supply.

These particles may be anything from cattle manure to animal carcasses to fallen leaves. The by-products of this interaction are highly toxic.

In theory, the chemicals disinfect the water, but the resulting "disinfection by-products" or "DBPs" are 1000 times more toxic than the decontaminants themselves.

At one time, chlorine was the primary additive in drinking water. Most treatment facilities, however, now use chloramine, which is a combination of chlorine and ammonia.

Chloramine cannot be removed from water by distilling, boiling, or outgassing (allowing the water to stand uncovered overnight.) Three of the disinfection by-products with which the report was most concerned are

Part I: Age 0-6 Months, Breast Milk or Formula

- trihalomethanes – associated with bladder cancer as well as gestational and developmental problems in children

- volatile organic compounds – which damage the central nervous system and irritate mucous membranes

- haloacetic acids – connected to liver disease, retardation of growth, low birth weight, neurological defects, and sperm toxicity

Some experts warn pregnant women against showering in water treated with chloramine because the disinfection by-products are absorbed through the skin.

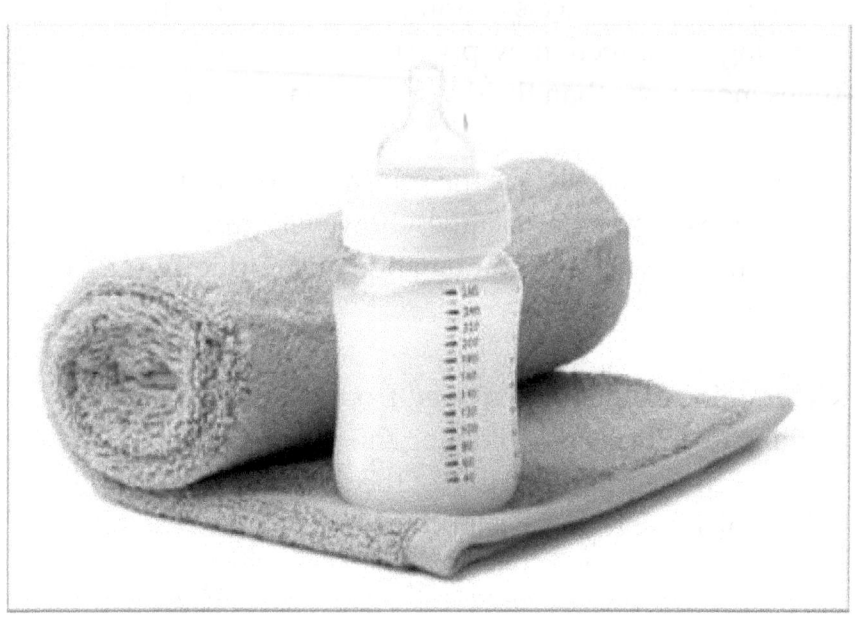

Part I: Age 0-6 Months, Breast Milk or Formula

This is all sufficiently frightening, however there is more. The report actually detected a total of 116,000 man-made chemicals in the municipal water supplies tested, including pharmaceuticals flushed into the sewers.

It is no easy matter to find chemical free water, since bottled water companies have been caught in the act of selling tap water and labelling it as "spring fed" or "all natural."

Premium Bottles

So-called "premium" bottles mimic the natural shape of the human breast. They are made of polycarbonate, but are certified to be free of BPA.

Since the nipple is incorporated in the design of the bottle rather than a separate unit, premium bottles are easier to clean.

You will, however, be faced with changing premium bottles according to a scheme of "flow rate" according to four age steps: birth to 3 months, 3-6 months, 6-9 months, 9 or more months.

Stainless Steel

Stainless steel baby bottles are relatively new on the market. They are not inexpensive, but the material is believed by many to be cleaner and free of potentially toxic chemicals. These hourglass shaped bottles are typically sold in sizes of 5-9 ounces / 148 – 266 mil with varying flow rates.

Part I: Age 0-6 Months, Breast Milk or Formula

Buying Baby Bottles

Your first lesson in just how stubborn a baby can be may come when you buy what you regard to be the "perfect" baby bottle and your child hates it!

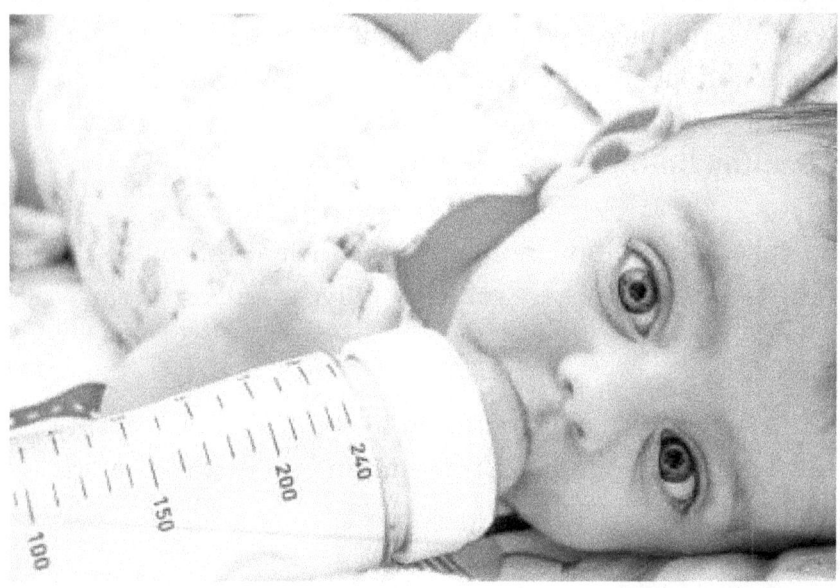

Bottles and nipples come in all sizes and styles, so be prepared to go through some experimentation before you find what your infant likes and will reliably use. The primary guiding factor in your selection really should be materials.

In July 2012 in the United States, the Food and Drug Administration banned the use of bisphenol A or "BPA" in baby bottles and "sippy" cups. (BPAs have been banned in Europe since March 2011.)

Part I: Age 0-6 Months, Breast Milk or Formula

To make certain the product you are buying does not contain this chemical, don't buy plastics marked with the number "7" or opt for old-fashioned glass bottles.

Bottle Types

In terms of shape and size, there are many types of baby bottles available, starting with the iconic "standard" and running the gamut to the newer aluminum bottle that looks like a baby thermos!

Standard

Standard bottles have the classic shape we all think about when we hear the phrase "baby bottle." They typically hold 8-9 ounces, but can be found in a range of sizes from 4-11 ounces.

These bottles are easy to fill and hold. Most breast pumps and bottle warmers were designed with this shape of bottle in mind. Standard bottles are available in glass or plastic.

Angle Neck

Angle neck baby bottles facilitate being held at a 45 degree angle to allow milk to collect efficiently around the nipple. This means your child will swallow less air.

It's also possible to feed your baby with one of these bottles in a slightly more upright position, reducing the chance of fluid collecting in the ear canals.

Part I: Age 0-6 Months, Breast Milk or Formula

Most are outfitted with a vent in the base to help keep bubbles out of the mixture and to facilitate cleaning. The only drawback to the angle neck format is that it can be difficult to fill.

Wide Neck

Wide neck baby bottles are somewhat shorter and broader across than standard bottles. They are also available in plastic and glass. Supposedly a wider bottle feels more "breast-like" to the infant, and may be most appropriate for infants fed a combination of breast milk and formula.

Disposable Liner

These bottles are the middle ground between glass and plastic bottles. The outer shell is reusable, but the inner, pouch-like liner is discarded after each feeding.

The primary concern with these bottles is whether or not the liners are indeed free of BPAs. Although the liners, which collapse during the feeding, help to prevent your infant from ingesting air, they are also expensive over the long term.

Natural Flow

The design of these bottles is a two part central vent that acts like a straw. The idea is to eliminate the vacuum formed by the child's suckling to prevent air bubbles from forming.

Part I: Age 0-6 Months, Breast Milk or Formula

In theory, natural flow bottles reduce instances of colic and gas. The containers are available in both plastic and glass, but the straw attachment is difficult to clean without the included tiny brush.

How-To: Bottle Feeding Basics

It is recommended that you purchase glass baby bottles rather than plastic ones that may contain toxic bisphenol A and other chemicals that are released upon heating.

If you have never given a baby a bottle, you may want to find videos online or ask one of the nurses in the hospital to help you the first time you feed your baby.
Don't forget to burp you baby after a feeding to bring up any air the infant might have swallowed.

Step One:

Take all new bottles and nipples and submerge them in boiling water for a minimum of five minutes, allowing the items to dry on a clean towel. After this initial sterilization, the items can subsequently be run through a normal dishwashing cycle for cleaning.

Step Two:

Mix the formula following the instructions on the packaging precisely.

Part I: Age 0-6 Months, Breast Milk or Formula

Step Three:

Although there is no health-based rationale for heating formula, most babies prefer it if their bottles are placed in a bowl of warm water or simply under a stream a warm tap water. Never use boiling water or heat formula in the microwave.

Step Four:

Cradle the child in a partially upright position while supporting the baby's head. It is important not to bottle feed a baby that is lying down. The formula can accidentally run into the middle ear and cause an infection.

Tilt the bottle so that the formula is in the neck of the container and covering the nipple

Expect your baby to take 2-4 ounces / 59 – 118.3 mil) during the first few weeks every 2-4 hours. Do not try to get your child to finish a bottle. Let the infant take as much as it wants and then stop.

Burping Your Baby

When babies gulp down either breast milk or formula, they also swallow air that collects in the esophagus, especially if the child is young enough to lie down most of the time. This causes gas, and also leads to the child spitting up its food.

Part I: Age 0-6 Months, Breast Milk or Formula

Burping your child helps the baby to get rid of gas and hopefully to save off the regurgitation. For bottle fed babies, burp after the child has consumed 2-3 ounces / 59-89 mil). For breast fed children, burp the child when it's time to switch breasts and at the end of the feeding.

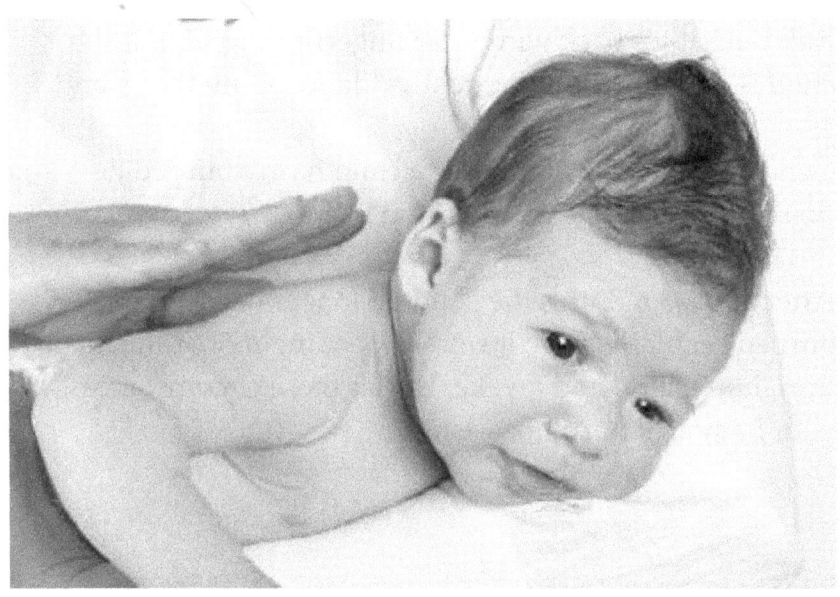

If it's clear, however, that your baby isn't spitting up much and really does not like it when you force him to stop for burping, it's okay to wait until the he signals he's had enough to eat.

To get those air bubbles up try one of these three positions:

- Put the baby on your shoulder.

- Sit the child up on your lap using a hand on the chest to support the chin.

Part I: Age 0-6 Months, Breast Milk or Formula

- Lay the baby face down across your lap with the head raised slightly on your thigh.

Regardless of the position, the baby's head should be just a little higher than the stomach.

Rub the baby's back with your fingertips or palm. If the child is on your shoulder gently "dance" with the infant.

Generally after 4-5 minutes if a child hasn't burped he doesn't need to and you can stop trying.

After age 2-3 months, the child no longer needs to be burped regularly since it's now spending more time in an upright position and awake. Under these circumstances, your baby will burp unassisted.

Part II – Age 6 Months - Introducing Solid Foods

Part II – Age 6 Months - Introducing Solid Foods

For the first 4-6 months of your baby's life, all the necessary nutrition for healthy growth and development comes from breast milk, formula, or a combination of the two. At 4-6 months, however, your child will start to develop an interest in solid food.

With this important dietary advancement, you not only have to consider what nutrients your child needs, but also to accurately judge the baby's readiness to eat solid foods.

Signs the Baby Wants Solids

Understand, however, that you don't have to start your child on solid food until 6 months of age, if you don't want to. Just make certain that you do not introduce solids any sooner than 17 weeks after your child's original due date.

Look for signs that your baby is ready to try new foods. For instance, you may be breastfeeding more often, the baby may seem hungry even after taking a full bottle, and the child may start to wake up hungry during the night.

A transition is definitely in the wings if the child is sitting up, holding its head up, and using a "palmar grasp" — holding on to things and bringing them to its mouth. Also, the baby will lose the reflex to stick out its tongue, which would force offered food away.

Basically a new level of communication is developing between you and your child around an evolving language

Part II – Age 6 Months - Introducing Solid Foods

of food. Most of the interpretation is left up to you, however!

Making the Move to Solids

If you think the baby is ready to try solids, mix up some rice cereal (the kind fortified with iron) and use formula or breast milk for the liquid. At this nutritional stage, foods fortified with iron are important because the child's iron levels have begun to drop.

As you progress through your child's transition to solids, you'll want to consider foods that are rich in iron, including:

- dark green vegetables
- legumes (beans)
- avocados
- brown rice
- cooked egg yolks
- meat

Infants and toddlers often suffer from iron deficiency. Feeding foods rich in Vitamin C will further guard against this problem, since Vitamin C aids in the absorption of dietary iron.

Rice cereal is a great starter food, not only because it contains iron, but also because when mixed with breast milk or formula, the cereal offers adequate amounts of calories, protein, carbohydrates, and fat.

Part II – Age 6 Months - Introducing Solid Foods

Recommended Nutrients Birth to 6 Months

Protein	13 grams
Iron	6 grams
Calcium	400 milligrams
Vitamin A	375 IU
Vitamin C	30 milligrams

After introducing rice, begin to concentrate on foods rich in both Vitamins C and A. Examples include deep orange and deep green vegetables, and apple sauce. Always add foods one a time and not in combination. After 3 days on the food, if no adverse reactions have surfaced, your child isn't allergic to the item.

Schedule for Introducing Solid Foods

4-6 Months	
single grain cereals	rice, then oatmeal, mixed with breast milk or formula and not sweetened with sugar
6-8 months	
strained or pureed fruit	prunes, applesauce, or pears, pureed in a blender or mashed, with a watery consistency then gradually thickened
7-8 months	
strained or pureed vegetables	carrots, squash, peas, potatoes, avocados; baked/boiled/steamed until soft when pureed with added breast

Feeding Baby

Part II – Age 6 Months - Introducing Solid Foods

	milk/formula/water; gradually thicken in consistency
sources of protein	cut up and pureed chicken, turkey, boneless fish, beans (black/pinto/red)
8-10 months	
begin mashing not pureeing	
add "finger food"	oat cereal pieces, teething crackers, small pieces of whole grain pasta
in small amounts	yogurt, cottage cheese, small bites of cheese
the same food you're eating	cut in small chunks

When you're certain that your child doesn't have any food allergies, you can feed 2-3 different items per meal. This not only ensures that the baby's dietary and caloric needs are being met, it also gives your baby an enjoyable amount of variety.

If the baby rejects a new food, just take it away and don't force the issue. A few days later, try again. If you coax the child, or worse yet coerce it to eat something, it's likely the infant will refuse the food for good. With no pressure, however, babies often will accept a food they initially refused to touch.

Your baby's first few meals of "real" food will just be tiny exploratory tastes. Don't worry, babies are very good about communicating their preferences. Once you have identified

Part II – Age 6 Months - Introducing Solid Foods

the "favorites," you can start to experiment with different combinations.

Choking

Choking is a significant hazard in children from birth to age five. So long as your child is coughing, he is not truly choking. Coughing is the body's natural attempt to repel a foreign object lodged in the throat.

Encourage your child to cough, and do not attempt to remove anything from the throat unless you can actually see the object. Attempts at retrieval risk pushing the item farther into the airway.

Take the following precautions against choking:

- Always supervise your child during meals.

- Keep your child seated during meals. Do not let the baby lie down, walk, run, or play while eating.

- Encourage your child to take small bites and to chew thoroughly.

Be careful about giving your child nuts unless they are ground in a food processor, and be careful to spread sticky foods like peanut butter in thin layers only.

It is highly recommended that all parents take courses in the proper administration of infant and child CPR.

Part II – Age 6 Months - Introducing Solid Foods

Vegetarian, Vegan and Gluten Free Cooking

Feeding your baby a vegetarian or vegan diet can be a healthy choice so long as you carefully plan meals to ensure that all nutrients are included. Being gluten-free may be a matter of necessity, depending on the child's sensitivities.

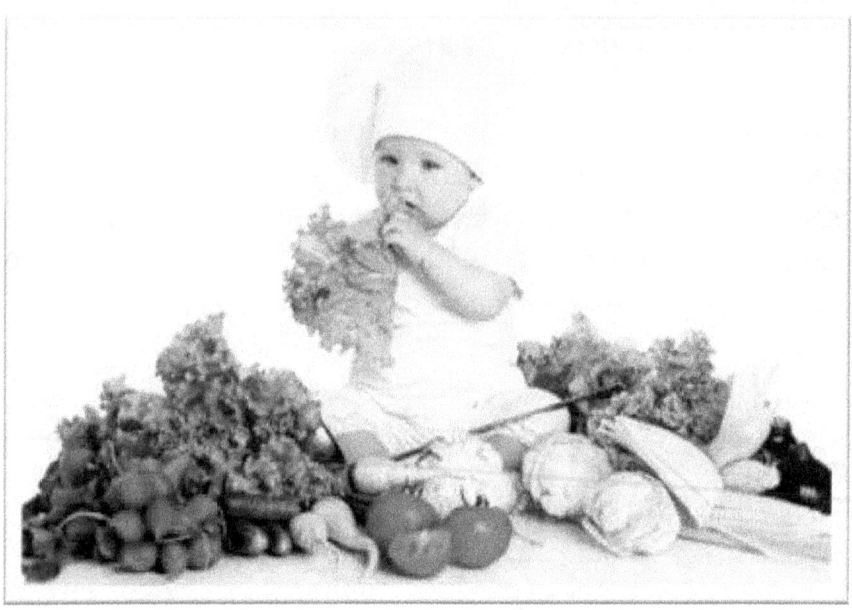

Designing a lacto-ovo vegetarian diet for an infant is easier than a strict vegan diet that completely avoids the consumption of any animal products. A vegan diet should not be undertaken without proper planning and education.

A gluten-free diet eliminates grains that contain the protein gluten including wheat, barley, rye, and triticale. In people who are gluten sensitive, exposure to gluten can cause severe gastrointestinal distress.

Part II – Age 6 Months - Introducing Solid Foods

If sufficiently severe, this sensitivity can actually manifest as Celiac Disease. Reactions to gluten can show up at any stage of a person's life.

Typically gluten sensitivity in infants will not surface until after 10 months. Before that time, children are not fed grains with gluten because those items are typically harder to digest.

Watching for Food Allergies

Be aware of any symptoms that might signal the presence of a food allergy including:

- rashes anywhere on the body
- loose stools
- diarrhea
- vomiting
- hives
- runny nose
- irritability
- gassiness
- labored breathing
- swelling of the lips, tongue, or face
- tightening / closure of the throat

Remember that there is a difference between a food allergy and food intolerance. If your child is exhibiting gastrointestinal symptoms only, you're likely dealing with

Part II – Age 6 Months - Introducing Solid Foods

a food intolerance. The most common food allergies are to the following items:

- eggs
- milk
- peanuts
- tree nuts (cashews and walnuts)
- shellfish
- fish
- soy
- wheat
- chocolate or cocoa
- citrus fruits or juices (orange, lime, grapefruit, and lemon)
- strawberries

Also beware of thickening agents, dyes and artificial colors, and preservatives.

Do not give honey to children under one year of age. Honey contains spores of the bacteria responsible for botulism, which is potentially deadly to infants.

Where to Feed the Baby

If your child can sit up unaided, place the infant in a high chair with pillows on the side for extra support if necessary. Always use the safety straps!

Part II – Age 6 Months - Introducing Solid Foods

For children still a little wobbly with sitting up, place the baby upright in your lap. Cradle the child's head in your arm. You can also place the child in its infant carrier set in the upright position.

Considering Baby Food in Jars

Contrary to what baby food manufacturers would have you believe, baby food in jars is not a nutritional halmark, nor is it superior to what you can prepare yourself at a much lower cost.

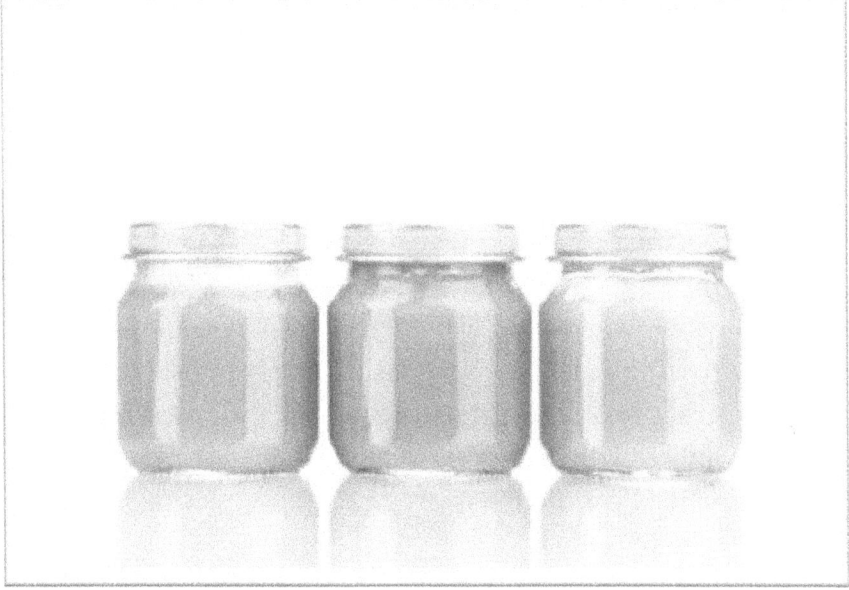

Most commercial baby food is diluted with substances like water and thickening agents, including flour and chemically modified starches that have no nutritional value.

Part II – Age 6 Months - Introducing Solid Foods

You're paying for fillers that don't provide superior nutrition and that may open your child up to sensitivities to substances like gluten and MSG.

With a blender or food processor, you can do just as well on your own. In many instances, you can get your child's food to the right consistency just by mashing it with a fork!

If you do buy baby food in jars, read the label carefully. Be forewarned that you may need a magnifying glass to do this no matter how well you see. Items you definitely want to avoid giving your child include:

- added sugar
- modified food starch
- flours including rice and wheat among others

When you buy a single food jar, it should contain nothing but the specified food and water. Good brand choices include:

- Growing Healthy, which is expensive but nutritious
- Gerber and Heinz meat/vegetable and meat/fruit combos, which don't contain fillers
- Earth's Best, which is organic (although this is not verified)

Definitely stay away from infant desserts that will only get your child's sweet tooth going. Use plain fruit instead or unsweetened apple sauce.

Part II – Age 6 Months - Introducing Solid Foods

REMEMBER, until your child reaches one year of age, the baby should still be drinking at least 20 ounces of breast milk or formula daily. Don't decrease these feedings!

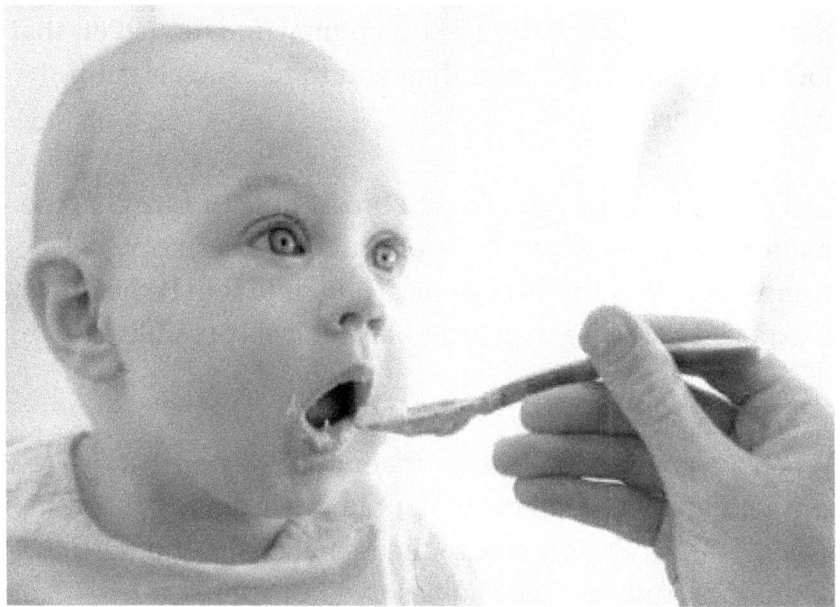

As long as you follow this rule, and offer your child a good variety of grains, fruits, and vegetables, the baby's nutritional needs will be met.

Deciding on Organic Foods

The term "organic" is generally accepted to refer to foods that are grown in the absence of pesticides, herbicides, fungicides, fertilizers, growth hormones, and antibiotics. Unfortunately, organics are often cost prohibitive for struggling young parents.

Part II – Age 6 Months - Introducing Solid Foods

Should You Buy Organic Produce?

Buying organic food that is as free as possible of pesticides, fertilizers, and all other chemicals is the foundation of homemade organic baby food. You may find, however, that locating organics is harder than you think, and certainly more expensive.

Just as with the decision to feed breast milk or formula, the matter or organics is an issue of choice. You can opt to go completely or partially organic. Your child will be healthier if exposed to the least amount of chemicals possible early in life.

When a baby eats foods with chemicals, they are being exposed to a far greater extent, pound per pound, than an adult. This is not only due to their smaller size, but also the amount of fruits and vegetables they consume.

Pesticides and other chemicals overload the liver, while hormones interfere with the child's natural development. Overall, foods with no chemicals that have not been genetically modified in any way are best for babies.

Organic baby food is prepared with the normal procedures. Cook by steaming or boiling. Then create the correct soft consistency with a masher, blender, or even a large fork. Use breast milk or formula to make the mixture as thick or thin as you like.

Part II – Age 6 Months - Introducing Solid Foods

There is no need to add salt to the food. Babies don't crave it, and you don't want to encourage salt consumption early in life.

Organic foods are not necessarily more nutritious that non-organics, so do not feel you're exposing your child to danger if you don't use or can't afford these items.

It is a good idea however to selectively purchase the following products as organics since both the U.S. Department of Agriculture and the Federal Food and Drug Administration rate them highest in pesticide content. (Note that the list is ordered from highest to lowest amount of pesticide present.)

- peaches
- strawberries
- apples
- cherries
- sweet bell peppers
- kale/collard greens
- celery
- potatoes
- nectarines
- imported grapes
- blueberries
- spinach

The level of pesticides present in these items cannot be reduced by simply washing them.

Part II – Age 6 Months - Introducing Solid Foods

The following "Clean 15" returns almost no evidence of pesticide presence, and are safe to purchase as non-organics:

- asparagus
- avocado
- cabbage
- cantaloupe
- sweet corn
- eggplant
- grapefruit
- kiwi
- mango
- mushroom
- onions
- papaya
- pineapple
- sweet peas
- sweet potatoes

Equipment Considerations

Most standard well-equipped kitchens will have everything you need to prepare and store your child's food, but consider the following as a basic checklist.

- food grinder
- food processor
- blender
- chopping knife and paring knife

Part II – Age 6 Months - Introducing Solid Foods

- tempered glass or plastic cutting boards
- kitchen scissors
- measuring cups and spoons
- assorted microwave safe bowls with lids
- small containers with lids for leftovers
- assorted microwave safe baking dishes
- small to medium frying pans and sauce pans with lids
- instant-read meat thermometer
- timer
- potato masher
- vegetable brush and peeler
- rubber spatulas
- small sieve or strainer

You'll also want feeding cups, weaning bowl(s) (with or without suction cups), and a weaning spoon.

A few things you'll want to keep on hand at all times include:

- unsweetened applesauce
- canned fruit nectar (without added sugar)
- frozen vegetables
- natural pasta sauce (without added sugar)
- whole grain pasta
- low-sugar whole grain cereal
- natural chicken broth (low sodium)
- oatmeal

Part II – Age 6 Months - Introducing Solid Foods

- brown rice
- peanut butter, almond butter, other nut butters
- pure canned pumpkin

This list is certainly not all inclusive, and should be individually tailored to your child's particular preferences.

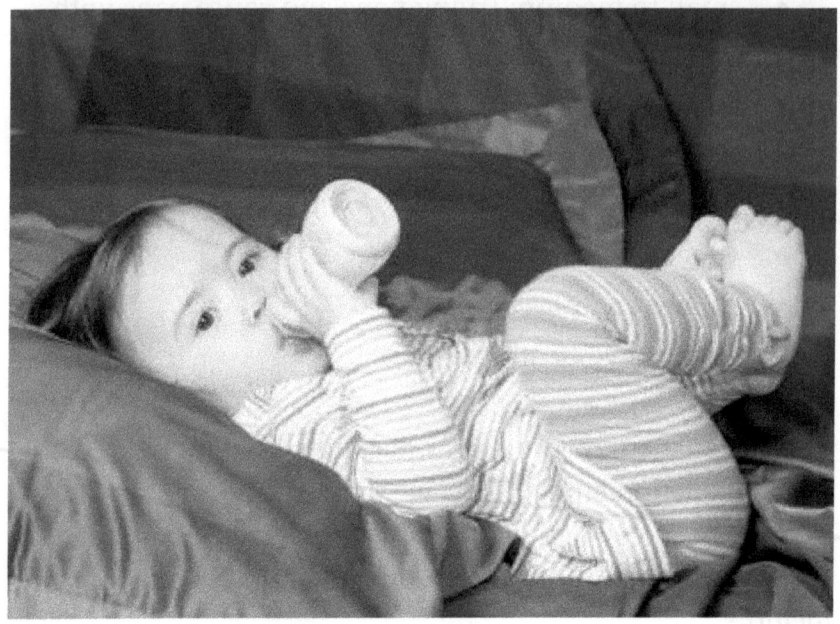

Storing Homemade Baby Food

One of the easiest ways to store large batches of baby food in the freezer is to use ice cube trays and simple freezer bags.

Each of the individual compartments in the tray is approximately one ounce / 30 mil. Spoon the food you have prepared into the compartments and then pop out the servings once they are frozen.

Part II – Age 6 Months - Introducing Solid Foods

Transfer the food cubes to freezer bags, which will take up less room in the freezer than the trays themselves. Label the bags, always including the preparation date and the name of the food. All frozen baby food looks remarkable alike!

When you are ready to use the food, simply take out the items you need and allow them to thaw.

Although you can store baby food in the refrigerator, it must be consumed within 48 hours or bacteria will build up. Never store baby "left overs." Only food that has not been touched should go into the refrigerator.

Do not microwave any type of baby food. The items get much hotter than you expect, and due to the uneven nature of the heating, there may be some "pockets" that are not enough to be dangerous.

Your baby's first meals should be mainly pureed and have more liquid content, gradually progressing to a more "mashed" texture. Each child is different, but typically this transition occurs over a 2 month period.

Be sure that the fruits you choose are ripe and soft. Wash everything, and remove any seeds or pits that might be present.

Liquid is still being derived primarily from breast milk or formula with no more than 1/2 cup / .24 liters, of diluted juice per day.

Part II – Age 6 Months - Introducing Solid Foods

Everything you offer your child should be lukewarm or at warm temperature. Foods are introduced one at a time to judge the child's reaction both in terms of taste preference and tolerance.

Starter foods should be very simple. Unsweetened applesauce, for instance, should be a staple of your pantry.

You can never go wrong with a combination of ground rolled oats, a pureed fruit and liquid in the form of breast milk or formula. Alternate this with pureed vegetables and you will have success! You can prepare things like:

A Grain and Fruit

1/4 cup ground rolled oats
1/2 cup breast milk/formula
1/3 ripe banana or cooked pear or cooked apple

The ratio of liquid to cereal should always be 2 to 1, regardless of the measurement system you are using.

Bring the cereal and liquid to a boil while stirring. Be sure the oats have been ground to a fine consistency.

When the cereal is boiling, remove the pan from the heat and cover. Let the cereal stand for 5 minutes before adding the soft fruit.

Use additional breast milk or formula if thinning is needed.

Part II – Age 6 Months - Introducing Solid Foods

Pureed Sweet Potatoes

Place an unwrapped, washed sweet potato in a pre-heated 400 F oven for 30-50 minutes. Allow the potato to cool before peeling off the skin and cutting the remainder in chunks and pureeing in the blender.
Each sweet potato should yield about 3 servings.

Sweet potatoes are rich in beta-carotene. Just 2 tablespoons of the puree per day will give your baby the recommended 500 mcg.

This same simple method can be used for butternut squash, which is also an excellent source of beta-carotene.

By 8 months, your child will be ready for soft, chunky foods that will encourage better chewing. Very ripe fruits, beans, and carrots are good choices.

At 9 months, your son or daughter will be eating 3 times a day, and should be encouraged to feed themselves and to touch their food.

This is the stage to start incorporating poultry, beef, and ham for protein content. Hardboiled or scrambled eggs 2-3 times per week will also add even more nutrition and calorie content.

By 10 months, the baby will be enjoying 3-4 meals per day and will be having what the family is eating. Talk to your child about what you are feeding him.

Part II – Age 6 Months - Introducing Solid Foods

Name foods and smile so that the baby associates a happy, enjoyable time with each item. It's a strategy that can make the difference if your child is being a bit fussy about a particular food. It doesn't hurt if you eat the food as well.

In another month, you have a toddler on your hands who is happily eating solids. There are definite likes and dislikes in place, and you can start experimenting with greater variety.

Let's face it, your child will have his or her own preferred foods and some will be more pleasing than others. Your baby is not necessarily being fussy, just deciding what's tasty and what isn't.

Continue to introduce new foods consistently. Even an unappealing food, especially if paired with a preferred food, can make all the difference in changing your child's mind.

A Word About Food Safety

Always practice good rules of food safety. Keep a clean kitchen both in terms of your food preparation area, but also your cooking utensils and food storage containers.

Be mindful of temperature. Discard any food that has been allowed to sit out at room temperature for an hour or more.

Wash your hands before and after handling each food item, especially poultry. Wash all fruits and vegetables under running water for at least 30 seconds.

Part III - Your Child's Nutritional Needs

The body requires nutrients for metabolism and growth. Many explanations of dietary needs attempt to focus on precise calculations of individual nutrients without considering the broader benefits to be had from whole foods offered in a wide variety.

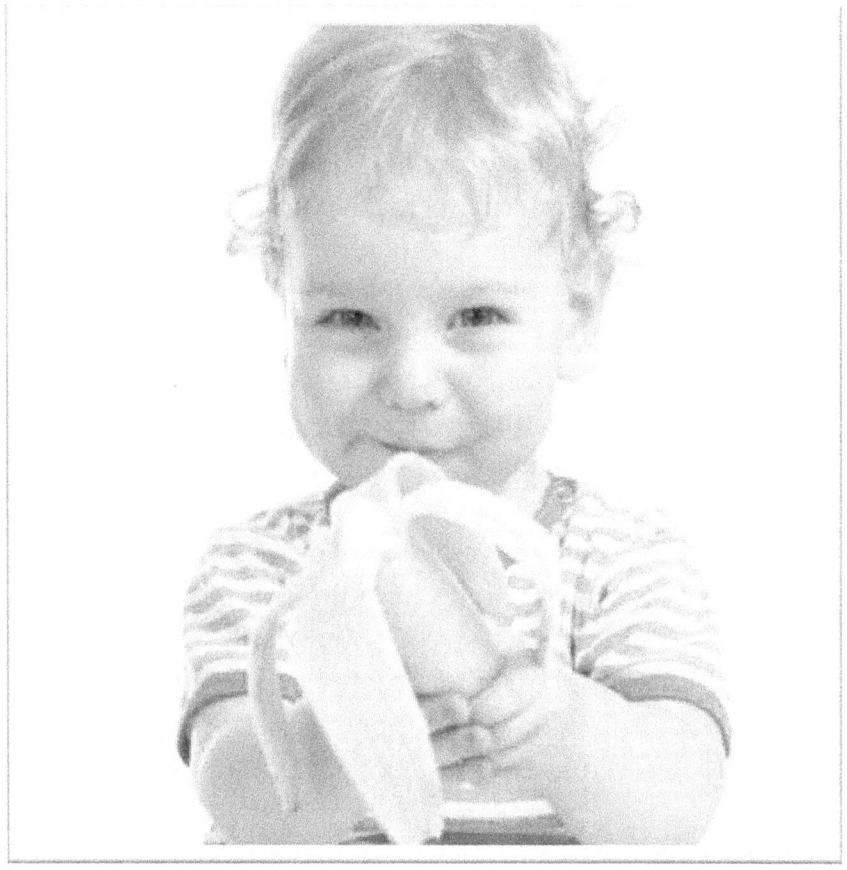

The relationship between the food we eat and our general health is intricate and far reaching. What you feed your

Part III - Your Child's Nutritional Needs

child in the first 24 months of life establishes your baby's primary relationship to food.

The more variety you can encourage your son or daughter to accept, the stronger their nutritional profile will be throughout life.

Simple and Complex Carbohydrates

We hear a great deal for and against carbohydrates from diet gurus, but far too often we lose sight of the fact that these "macronutrients," which our bodies require in large amounts, are the primary fuel for the human "engine."

Carbohydrates are easily digestible sources of energy required for the proper functioning of the brain and central nervous system, the gastrointestinal system, and our muscles. They are comprised of chains of sugar, and are classified as either "simple" or "complex."

Simple carbohydrates have one or two chains of sugar while complex carbohydrates have three or more. Think of simple carbohydrates as "sweet." They deliver a quick energy "hit." Complex carbohydrates are starchy and digest slowly, allowing for a supply of energy that is gradually released over time.

Foods that are rich in lactose, sucrose, fructose, and glucose are simple carbohydrates. These include dairy products, vegetables, and fruits.

Part III - Your Child's Nutritional Needs

Many processed and refined foods contain simple carbohydrates as sweetening agents. This is why sweet soda drinks and candy bars are often thought of as "fast energy" foods.

Simple carbohydrates in the form of refined sugars of this type are, however, empty calories. They don't deliver any benefit in terms of fiber content, vitamins, or minerals.

A perfect example is high fructose corn syrup, which is held to be responsible for the epidemic of obesity in America that extends to very young children.

A well-balanced diet should be as free of refined sugars as possible. They not only contribute to weight gain, but are also major contributors in the spread of diabetes, liver disease, and cardiovascular disease.

Complex carbohydrates are found in whole grains, starchy vegetables, and legumes (including peas, peanuts, lentils, and beans.) Often refined foods have been stripped of these natural nutrients and then "enriched."

Soluble and Insoluble Fiber

Fiber is another macronutrient specifically derived from plants. It is present in our diet in two forms, soluble and insoluble. They function differently, but each is important.

Because soluble fiber absorbs water, it makes the stomach feel full and slows down digestion. If you eat a lot of soluble fiber, you also need to drink adequate amounts of

Part III - Your Child's Nutritional Needs

water, or constipation will result. Infants don't need additional water because they get the hydration they need from breast milk.

Examples of soluble fiber include: seeds and nuts, oats, legumes, broccoli, onions, sweet potatoes, carrots, apples, oranges, pears, and plums.

Insoluble fiber is bulky and moves quickly through the digestive system, speeding up the removal of waste. A healthy amount of insoluble fiber serves as a natural laxative and enhances the function of the digestive system.

The insoluble fiber group includes white potatoes, dark leafy vegetables, avocados, whole grains, tomatoes, grapes, raisins, and bananas.

Complete and Incomplete Proteins

Protein serves multiple functions in the body, supplying energy, and contributing to the growth of tissues. It enhances immune function, contributes to the production of hormones, and protects lean muscle mass.

Proteins are typically more satisfying than carbohydrates, staving off feelings of hunger for longer periods of time.

Humans derive 20 amino acids from food. Of those, nine cannot be made by our bodies and are thus termed "essential."

Part III - Your Child's Nutritional Needs

- histidine
- isoleucine
- lysine
- methionine
- phenylalanine
- threonine
- tryptophan
- valine

Proteins are divided into two categories: complete and incomplete.

Complete proteins contain all of the essential amino acids. These foods include beef, fish, lamb, and poultry as well as dairy products, eggs, and soybeans.

Incomplete proteins contain fewer than the complete 9 essential amino acids, or have one of these substances in insufficient quantities to meet the recommended levels.

Typically proteins derived from plant-based sources are incomplete, requiring complementary items offered throughout the day. Complete combinations would include:

- corn and beans
- rice and beans
- wheat toast and peanut butter

When working with a primarily plant-based diet, variety is the key to ensuring daily amino acid levels are met.

Part III - Your Child's Nutritional Needs
Saturated, Unsaturated, and Trans Fats

Fat is necessary for normal development and growth and are an important caloric source for both infants and toddlers.

During the first two years of life it's important not to limit fat intake so long as the sources are natural and not manmade (trans fats.) Fats assist in the growth of both the body and the brain. There are three types: saturated, unsaturated, and trans fats.

Use melting point as a baseline to distinguish which fat you're using. A substance that stays solid at room temperature, like butter, and has a relatively high melting point is a saturated fat.

Something like olive oil that is liquid at room temperature with a low melting point is an unsaturated fat.

Trans fats, on the other hand, are altered unsaturated fats. They are processed to make them more stable and essentially more solid at room temperature.

Animal sources are primarily saturated fats, with the exception of some items like coconut oil and butter and palm oil. These are the so-called "bad" fats because they are linked to cardiovascular disease and high cholesterol in adults.

Fish, nuts, and seeds are typically "good" or unsaturated fats, and can actually lower blood pressure and mitigate the risk of cardiovascular disease by increasing HDL cholesterol.

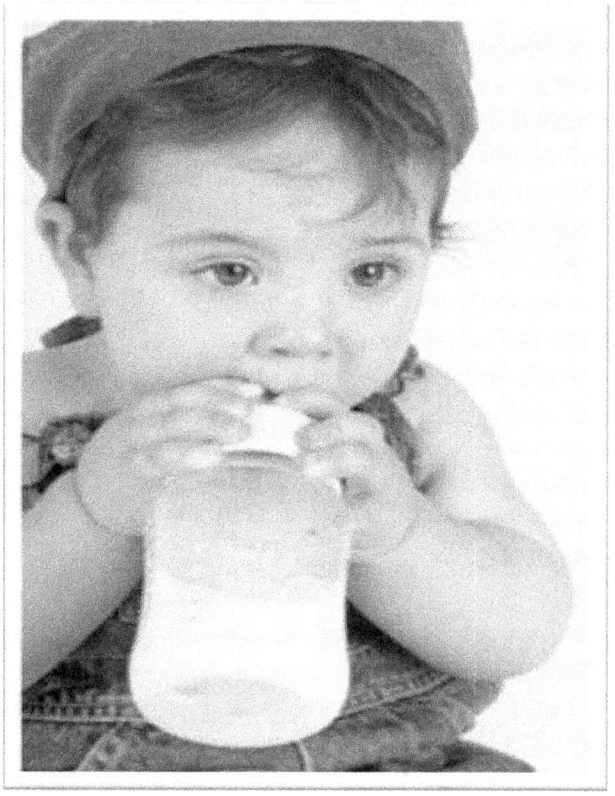

Unsaturated fats that are not synthesized by humans are called "essential fatty acids." There are two categories, omega-3 and omega-6.

You need both in balance since omega-6s in isolation increase inflammation and blood clotting while omega-3s counteract those effects while enhancing immune function and cell growth. As a rule, the Western diet is higher in omega-6s than in omega-3s.

Trans fats are found in processed foods and commercially baked items. Things like margarine and vegetable shortening are full of trans fats, which raise levels of "bad" LDL cholesterol.

Vitamins and Minerals

Vitamins and minerals are termed "micronutrients" because our body needs them in smaller amounts. These substances do a variety of things like aiding the formation of red blood cells or strengthening our bones and teeth.

The essential vitamins are: A, B in all its forms, C, D, E, and K, while the important minerals are iron, sodium, potassium, magnesium, calcium, zinc, selenium, iodine, and phosphorous.

The best nutritional approach to vitamin and mineral content is to derive these substances from a balanced diet, not from supplementation.

This fact highlights just how important the concept of "balance" really is. For instance, vitamins A, D, E, and K are fat soluble. Without adequate amounts of dietary fat, these nutrients don't work well in the body.

The good news is that fat soluble vitamins don't have to be eaten every day, because they are stored in the body's tissues and eliminated rather slowly. Food-based sources for the fat soluble vitamins include:

Part III - Your Child's Nutritional Needs

Vitamin A	Animal and dairy products, liver, egg yolks, and fish oils. Carrots, sweet potatoes, cantaloupe, mangoes, apricots, dark green leafy vegetables.
Vitamin D	Egg yolks, salmon and other fatty fish, liver, and fortified dairy products.
Vitamin E	Dark green leafy vegetables, avocados, wheat germ, vegetable oils, nuts, and seeds.
Vitamin K	Dark green leafy vegetables including spinach, chard, parsley and kale, as well as asparagus, peas, and broccoli. Also cashew nuts, pumpkin seeds, and pistachios.

The body does not store water soluble vitamins, which includes the B vitamins and Vitamin C. These nutrients must be consumed on a regular basis.

B Vitamins (B1, B2, B3, B5, B6, B7, B9, B12*)	legumes, seeds and nuts, whole grains, eggs and dairy, meats and fish, molasses, nutritional yeast, vegetables, fruits
Vitamin C	citrus fruits, papaya, mangoes, cantaloupe, strawberries, red and green sweet bell peppers, spinach, chard, kale, tomatoes, broccoli, cauliflower, turnips, Brussels sprouts

*Of the B vitamins, B12 is the only one derived from animal products. For this reason, vegans must be careful about developing a B12 deficiency.

Part III - Your Child's Nutritional Needs

Iron

A baby is born with enough iron in its system to last 6 months, after which time external sources of iron are needed. Iron deficiency or anemia is the most common of all nutritional issues in babies, leading to weakness, fatigue, and a pale skin tone.

Iron's role in the body is to carry oxygen. Both animal and plant-based foods provide iron. "Heme" iron is derived from meats and is more readily absorbed by the body, while non-heme iron comes from plants.

In diets that emphasize non-heme iron, eating foods rich in Vitamin C at the same meal will enhance iron absorption and increase the dietary benefit. However, if the same non-heme food is mixed with dairy products or other sources calcium, the benefit of the iron will be lost.

Calcium

Typically, infants and babies get all the calcium they need from breast milk and/or formula. As the consumption of these liquid sources begins to decrease around one year, ensuring the presence of adequate dietary calcium becomes important.

Not only is calcium essential for building strong bones and teeth, it is also necessary for digestive, muscle, and heart health.

Part III - Your Child's Nutritional Needs

Good sources of calcium include eggs and dairy products, nuts and seeds, and dark green leafy vegetables.

Part III - Your Child's Nutritional Needs

The Scoop on Poop

Most parents look to the contents of the diaper to get a sense of how well their infant or toddler is handling what they're being fed. Understanding what you are seeing is not, however, quite as simple as you might think.

Meconium

This newborn fecal matter often startles new parents because it looks distinctly like sticky motor oil with a greenish tint. It is the remains of what your child ingested while in the womb, including amniotic fluid. Thankfully, it doesn't have a strong odor, so you will have to be more vigilant about checking for diaper changes.

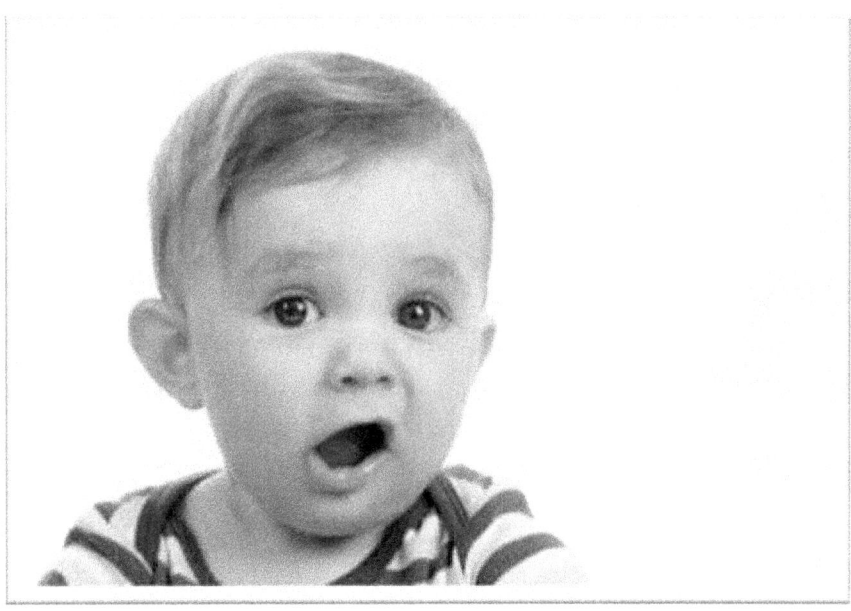

The Scoop on Poop

Transitional Stools

By 2-4 days, a child's stools began to lighten in color and to be less sticky. The greenish tint is still present. Now the baby is eating either breast milk or formula, and stools with this constancy and color mean that digestively, everything is going according to plan.

Breastfed Babies

Babies that are fed only breast milk pass stools that are soft in consistency and slightly green to yellow in tint. Some people say that the fecal matter resembles mustard. It may or may not be flecked. There is only minimal odor.

If a breast-fed child's stools are bright green, the infant is getting too much "fore milk," the lower calories milk that is first released during a feeding rather than the richer "hind milk." This could indicate the baby is not being allowed to feed long enough on each breast.

Formula Fed Babies

Babies that are fed formula only pass stools that are roughly the color and consistency of peanut butter, although the shades can range from tan to green-brown. There will be more odor than with children that are breastfed.

The Scoop on Poop

Blackish Stools

If your baby is receiving an iron supplement, dark green to black stools are normal. If, however, your child is not receiving iron, black stools could indicate the presence of blood and should be evaluated.

Solid Foods

Once your baby begins to receive solid food, the stools become thicker in consistency and are brown to dark brown. The odor also increases.

The occasional bit of undigested food is nothing to be worried about, especially if your child is not yet chewing well. If, however, this goes on constantly, consult with your doctor.

Problem Poops

Babies that have diarrhea pass runny stools that are more liquid than solid, and can range from yellow to green and brown. If your child is 3 months old or younger, call the doctor after 2-3 diapers.

Constipated babies pass hard stools that look like pebbles and may be tinged with blood. The child will appear uncomfortable when defecating. This often happens when a baby is being given solids for the first time.

Consult with your doctor, who may recommend water, pear, or prune juice.

The Scoop on Poop

If the feces are covered in streaks of mucous, an infection or allergy may be present. Your doctor should be the one to evaluate this problem if it continues for 2 days or more.

Blood in the feces is always a cause for concern. In normal feces, the blood may indicate a milk protein allergy, or in diarrhea, the presence of a bacterial infection.

Blackish blood that appears as flecks in the stools of breast fed babies indicates they are swallowing blood from the breast, meaning you are the one in need of attention

If you see anything in the diaper that is highly unusual and alarming, err on the side of caution and call the doctor. Thankfully such occurrences are rare, but they should never be ignored.

Part IV – 12 to 24 Months

Part IV – 12 to 24 Months

Toddlers don't grow as rapidly as babies. Infants can put on 3 inches / 7.62 cm every 3 months, whereas a toddler may grow 3-5 inches / 7.62 – 12.7 cm, over the course of a year. Nutrition remains critical, but you and your child are now moving into new territory.

Although your son or daughter will have a slower food intake in the second year of life, it will be based on increased levels of preference and independence.

Bottles will give way to cups, fingers will come into play, and the food choices will evolve significantly in variety and combination.

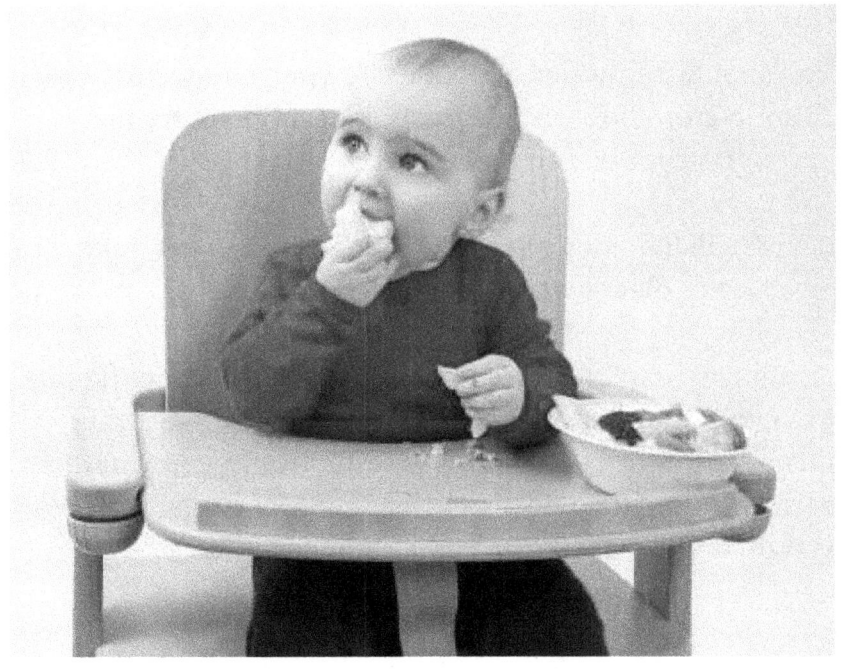

Part IV – 12 to 24 Months

Evolving Eating Skills

A toddler's eating skills are in a period of transition from 12-24 months. By 15 months, your little one will have mastered self-feeding with fingers and likely be progressing nicely with a spoon.

At first, your toddler may regard the spoon as more toy than tool. These are the months of the amazingly well-timed splatter. It's almost staggering how well a baby with a spoon can hit everything in range but his mouth!

You will be cleaning constantly. It's not a bad idea to put a mat down under your child's high chair. Some mothers bless the family pets that stand ever at the ready to assist with dropped and spilled food.

You should be cautious about using your canine or feline cleanup crew, however, as many human foods are not appropriate for our animal friends.

Beyond all that, however, Fido and Fluffy can get quite fat on a steady diet of whatever your toddler drops!

As soon as your child seems ready, offer him or her liquids in a cup rather than a bottle. They need to cultivate the manual dexterity to handle and drink from a cup, but this early introduction will also ease the future struggles when you do decide to take the bottle away for good.

Part IV – 12 to 24 Months

Scheduled Meals and Snacks

During the first year of life, your child ran the show in terms of feeding times. Now, it's appropriate to move toward more structured and routine meals and snacks. This change alone will make your life much easier, affording you a greater ability to plan and schedule.

It isn't necessary for your child to eat a great deal at any one meal. You are trying to accustom the toddler to the idea of regular, predictable times when food is to be offered. Your child will feel more secure on a regular schedule once they understand that the same thing is going to happen every day.

This is also the perfect time to begin modeling good eating habits for your child. As the toddler approaches age 2, they can eat whatever the family is having, gaining complete nutrition from high-quality foods offered in good variety.

How Much Food?

Toddlers need on average 1,000-1,400 calories a day. It's always important to use your own judgment and to take cues from your child on their levels of hunger and satisfaction.

The following targets are, however, a good starting point to work out appropriate daily intake in the second year of life:

Part IV – 12 to 24 Months

Whole Grains: 3 ounces. This is roughly equivalent to a slice of bread, a cup of cereal, or half a cup (US or UK) of rice.

Vegetables: 1 cup. Serve soft vegetables cut into small pieces and use a measuring cup.

Fruits: 1 cup. This is the equivalent of an 8-9 inch banana. Make sure the fruits are soft, and use a measuring cup.

Milk or Dairy: 2 cups. The recommended daily intake of milk can be a cup of milk or yogurt and 1.5-2 ounces / 43 – 57 grams, of a natural cheese.

Meats and Beans: 2 ounces. Divide this between an ounce / 28 grams, of meat, poultry or fish, a quarter of a cup of dried beans, and an egg (2 or 3 times a week.)

Children age 12-24 months should be given whole milk in order to benefit from the dietary fats, but in families with a history of cardiovascular disease and obesity, reduced fat (2%) or low-fat (1%) milk may be the better option.

Discuss the issue of milk with your doctor. Most children do not take readily to cow's milk because the taste is so different from breast milk or formula.

Mixing cow's milk with either of these liquids and increasing the amount slowly over time can ease the transition.

Part IV – 12 to 24 Months

If you have a child who does not like milk, or who cannot tolerate milk, you can explore other calcium-rich beverages like those made from soy. There are also calcium-fortified juices, breads, and cereals.

Many foods are naturally rich in calcium including beans, and dark green vegetables like broccoli, kale, and bok choy.

Teething

Some teeth will begin to appear as early as 4 months, but by age 3, all of the 20 primary teeth are in place. Dental care for your baby should begin as soon as the first teeth appear.

Teething babies can and do want to chew on anything to get some relief from the discomfort they are feeling. It's important to watch what your child is gnawing on during this period.

A cold, damp washcloth is a good option. Never leave a teething child alone with an object in their mouths, however, and be diligent about keeping the drool wiped off the chin so the skin won't become irritated.

Eating Practices

Between birth and age 5, children learn how to eat based on the culture to which they are exposed and the habits of their families.

If you as a parent are more worried about how much your child eats, rather than what is being consumed, you're

Feeding Baby

Part IV – 12 to 24 Months

working from an old-fashioned scarcity relationship with eating.

Quality counts much more than quantity when feeding your child. The last thing you want to do is encourage over eating early in life.

Instead of offering your child packaged, processed foods full of empty calories and packed with sugar, fat, and salt, help your son or daughter become accustomed to superior natural foods.

Don't serve a limited menu. It's not just genes that effects future chances of obesity, but also parenting styles. Today's children are at a greater risk for becoming overweight earlier in life than any generation before them.

Teach good eating habits by practicing them. Serve three meals a day and 2-3 planned snacks. Offer a fruit or vegetable at every meal, and don't label your child "picky." If you do, they'll wear the label proudly and to the extreme.

Focus your attention on your children at meal times, placing food before them without background distractions. A family that routinely eats in front of the television or computer will inevitably give in to mindless eating.

Help your child to craft a positive relationship with food now, and you will be giving a gift of better, healthier eating that will last a lifetime.

Recipes? Not Really

This is a "take the bull by the horns" moment. You really do not need a "recipe" to make baby food! While I was researching this book, I was somewhat confounded by a page online that offered a recipe for a "perfect" first food for a baby — an avocado.

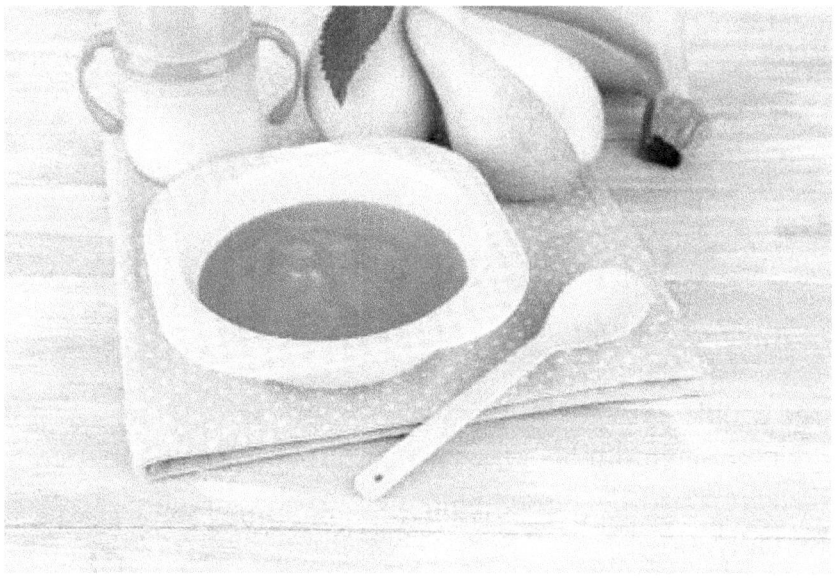

I don't disagree with that. Babies love avocados. But the recipe was essentially this:

- buy an organic avocado
- use a knife to peel the avocado
- mash the flesh up with a spoon
- feed to your child

It's not that I don't understand being a fearful cook. I never was one, but I have a friend who treats a recipe like a

Recipes? Not Really

chemistry experiment — everything must be measured just so or she's convinced the kitchen will blow up.

You need to be worried about consistency and quality.

At about six months of age babies start eating thin, liquid-based foods and work up to soft, pureed foods served in small bites. In many cases, you can "make" baby food by just take a fork and mashing something up.

That "recipe" might read:

- boil carrots until soft
- mash with a fork
- thin with breast milk or formula
- feed to your child

The problem here is that worried mothers think they must get precise amounts of this or that nutrient into their child on a set schedule. Surely this must involve a recipe? Actually, no.

The predominant "recipe" has one ingredient — variety.

Encourage your child to eat whole foods in variety, and don't worry so much about the process — or how disgusting you find the combinations your child loves.

Maybe you wouldn't eat unsweetened applesauce, mashed up avocado and oatmeal cereal at one meal, but your toddler loves the trio and bangs on the high chair for more. Great! Mash up another avocado!

Recipes? Not Really

Throughout this book, I've emphasized the need to continue using breast milk and formula even after you've introduced solids. I've talked about the value of various foods and suggested potential first foods.

You can take it from there! Really, you can. Don't be afraid for one minute to try. Puree whole fruits and vegetables. Label the items so you know what you're thawing out and serving. Improvise!

Many mothers get so wrapped up in perfection, they forget to have fun with their children. Have fun feeding your baby as well.

If you serve a combination of items to your child and he throws the stuff on the floor every single time, sooner or later you'll get the message he doesn't like those things.

Taste them yourself. If you think they're disgusting, perhaps your child does as well. There's a rather famous story told in my family about me and my mother's insistence that I eat turnips of all things as a toddler.

She kept cooking them. I kept throwing them all over the kitchen. Finally the day came when my extremely patient father said, "That's enough. She doesn't like them. She's made it very clear she doesn't like them. Stop trying to get her to eat them." To my certain knowledge, I have never eaten a turnip since.

You and your baby will work out your own "recipes." You will discover what your baby does and doesn't like,

Recipes? Not Really

especially as the child can begin to eat the things you're serving your family.

But in the first two years of life? Keep the consistency soft and concentrate on a healthy variety of whole foods — nothing processed. There's your recipe!

Afterword

Setting idealistic goals for yourself and for your child is part of being a parent. Time and circumstances have a way of wearing down those ideals. Just ask the last children born to large families. "Where are all the pictures of ME?" they demand indignantly.

Raising a child is hard work on all levels. You never get too tired to be worried about what your child is eating, however, especially when you look around at other children on the playground and in daycare facilities.

Obesity has slowly found its way into the youngest levels of our society, in part because the modern diet relies too heavily on processed foods filled with fat, salt, and sugar as well as chemical additives and now "genetically modified organisms."

Many of these substances have been scientifically proven to be addictive. When children begin eating them early in life, they find giving them up later on to be extremely difficult. You are not only charged with providing your child with good nutrition now, but with helping your son or daughter cultivate good eating habits that will last a lifetime. No wonder you're worried!

In this book I have tried to encourage parents to develop realistic and attainable goals, not perfection. I am, frankly, not a fan of perfection for the simple reason that it doesn't exist. It's a bludgeon with which exhausted and guilty parents beat themselves.

Afterword

Have you ever listened ruefully to a grandparent or other elderly relative observe sagely, "You ate dirt out of the garden at that age and it didn't kill you?" Well, the dirt in that garden wasn't full of pesticides and fertilizers, and the fruits and vegetables hadn't been genetically altered.

It's not as easy today as it was even 25 years ago to find healthy whole foods to feed your baby. That is, however, in my belief, the foundation of good nutrition. There is no reason to react in horror to the notion of making your own baby food.

It's actually much less expensive to buy a sweet potato, bake it, and mash it up with a little breast milk or formula than it is to buy pureed sweet potato baby food in a jar only to find out the mixture is filled with preservatives and other chemicals you don't want your child to eat.

At the same time, however, I am adamant that no two mothers are alike, nor are any two children identical. Family and work circumstances vary even more broadly.

Find what works for your life and home, and do that. Offer your child the best nutrition you are capable of obtaining, creating, and affording .

While I don't suggest sending your toddler out to eat dirt in the garden, healthy children are much more resilient than worried parents think they are.

Afterword

At the end of the day, your best is always good enough. You wouldn't have spent the time necessary to read this book if you didn't care about your child's nutritional needs — a fact about which you can remind them when they are teenagers and seem to think french fries are a food group.

One of my children is a vegetarian, another eats a very well rounded diet that includes meat, and I expect the third one to drop dead at any moment! They were all raised the same way, but they all have very different tastes.

Absolve yourself now. You are raising little individuals. While they are at home, you have some control over what they eat, but it won't last forever.

I gave my children a good foundation, and I actually have hope for the third one who recently told me, scornfully, "MOM! Of course I don't eat hot dogs! Do you know what they put IN those things?" He may have listened to me after all. I'll let you know.

Afterword

Relevant Websites

Parenting
www.parenting.com/baby/feeding

Parents
www.parents.com/baby/feeding/solid-foods/first-year-baby-feeding-guide

Dr. Greene
www.drgreene.com

Baby Center
www.babycenter.com/0_how-to-make-your-own-baby-food_1401482.bc

Homemade Baby Food Recipes
www.homemade-baby-food-recipes.com

Nurture Baby
www.nurturebaby.com

Sage Spoonfuls
www.sagespoonfuls.com/homemade

Kidspot Australia
www.kidspot.com.au/best-recipes/baby+3.htm

Martha Stewart BabyFood Recipes
www.marthastewart.com/267679/homemade-baby-food-basics

Relevant Websites

The Bump
http://www.thebump.com

HelloBee
http://boards.hellobee.com

Frequently Asked Questions

To completely understand all that is involved in meeting your child's nutritional needs, please read the entire text. The following frequently asked questions are provided as a quick reference only.

What kind of schedule should I follow for breastfeeding?

In the first month of life, newborns will nurse 8-12 times per day. Babies that are fed breast milk eat more often than those that receive formula because breast milk is easier for your child to digest and moves through his system more quickly.

From 1-2 months, feedings should stabilize at 7-9 times per day. Initially, the baby is completely in charge of the schedule, with feedings occuring every hour and a half to 3 hours.

As the child grows older, the frequency of feedings will decrease, and a more reliable schedule will develop. Newborns, however, should not go longer than four hours without a feeding nor should feedings be delayed overnight.

How do I count the feeding intervals? From the time the baby starts nursing or when the child stops?

Count the time from when the baby begins to nurse until the next feeding session begins. If you baby takes a feeding

Frequently Asked Questions

at 6 a.m., and then another at 8 a.m., the interval has been 2 hours.

How will I know when my baby is ready to eat?

Crying is not a reliable indication of hunger. The child may need to be changed, or could just want a comforting cuddle. When an infant is actually hungry, they open their mouths, stick their tongues out, and move their heads back and forth.

The baby may put their hands or their fists to their mouths, pucker their lips mimicking suckling, and nuzzle against your breast. Babies also exhibit behavior called the "rooting reflex," moving their mouths in the direction of something touching their cheek.

How long should a nursing session last?

There are many factors that affect the length of a feeding session. Until your milk supply has stabilized and you and your child are working together to get the positioning correct, times may vary. As the baby becomes more efficient, he may take as little as 5 minutes or as long as 20 minutes on each side.

How often should I alternate between breasts?

The goal is to give each breast the same amount of nursing time per day. This will keep the supply constant in each breast and prevent one or the other from becoming painfully engorged.

Frequently Asked Questions

There is no set rule about how long it will take a child to be satisfied on each breast. Do whatever works for you and your baby. Try alternating mid-way through the feeding and alternate which breast is offered first each time.

Some children do not like to switch breasts during feeding. Concentrate on comfort for both you and the child, and try to stick with the equal time per day recommendation.

Should I burp the baby during breast feedings?

Yes. Often when babies are switched from one breast to the other the movement causes them to burp anyway. When your nursing routine has been established, burp the child as often as you think is needed to help the baby be comfortable.

Babies that are spitting up often need more frequent burping. It's quite normal for a small amount of liquid to come up when a child is burped, but there should be no vomit. If this is occurring, check with your doctor to rule out any potential problems.

How will I know when my baby has had enough to eat?

If your baby is happy, content, and appears satisfied at the end of a feeding, the child has had enough to eat. Other indicators of adequate feeding include 4-6 wet diapers daily, regular bowel movements, good sleep, an alert manner when awake, and proper weight gain.

Frequently Asked Questions

Babies that aren't getting enough are fussy, have few daily diapers, seem to be hungry often, and aren't meeting their weight milestones. If you're concerned about how well your child is eating, talk to your doctor.

It may be necessary for your breastfeeding to be evaluated by a trained lactation specialist to correct issue with how the child is latching on, or other potential problems. Postnatal checkups always include taking the child's weight, so you can be assured of an accurate record.

For your own peace of mind, keep a breastfeeding journal. Write down the time and duration of the feeding session. Keep a record of diaper changes as well. It may be that your child is eating more than you realize.

What is normal to see in a baby's diaper?

At first, a newborn's stools are tarry and thick, but turn greenish yellow within 3-4 days of birth. For a more complete explanation of normal stools under various conditions, see the section of this book entitled, "The Scoop on Poop."

My baby seems to wants to nurse just for comfort. Should I allow this?

Once a baby has gotten enough to eat, he or she may stay at the breast for as long as an hour just for comfort. You can tell the difference by the lack of sucking action.

Frequently Asked Questions

Early in your baby's life, or if the infant is sick, allowing this kind of nursing for comfort is fine, but as the baby gets older, it can be problematic, especially if comfort nursing is required to get the baby to go to sleep at night or to take a nap.

You may opt to offer your child his or her own thumb to suck on, or perhaps give the baby a pacifier. The American Academy of Pediatrics recommends allowing babies to go to sleep with a pacifier to lower the risk of sudden infant death syndrome (SIDS).

Why does my baby seem to be hungrier than usual?

As babies grow they tend to eat more at each feeding and wait longer before asking for the next meal. At times, however, the child may seem hungrier, especially if they are going through a growth "spurt."

Such periods of rapid growth typically occur when babies are 7 to 14 days old, and then at 3, 4, and 6 months. Just follow your child's cues and, if necessary, increase the frequency of feedings.

What nutrients should my child get from solid foods?

That is an age-dependent question. In the earliest months of the transition to solid foods, babies are still getting most of their caloric content and nutritional value from either breast milk or formula.

Frequently Asked Questions

The solids they are receiving at this time are teaching them how to eat in a different way, but not replacing their primary nutritional mainstays. Moving forward, it's much better to concentrate on a variety of whole foods than on precise calculations of calories, vitamins, minerals, and proteins.

Be sure that your child is introduced to a wide range of foods to meet the necessary nutritional requirements as they fully transition to solids. The greater the choices present from whole food sources, the healthier your child's diet will be.

When should I start feeding meats?

Before 8 months of age, babies get all the protein they require from breast milk or formula. From 8 months forward, the child will begin to derive additional protein from both animal and vegetable sources.

Is fat important in my baby's diet?

Your baby needs fat to grow and for correct brain function. Fats help the body to absorb vitamins, and they serve as fuel for your child's rapid rate of development. Per gram, fats contain more calories than either protein or carbohydrates.

Just as a point of comparison, when the water is removed from breast milk, what is left is primarily fat. This is not an issue of worrying about your child being overweight. That

Frequently Asked Questions

concern may come later. Now you're worried about fueling that rapidly growing engine!

How many calories should my baby have?

Just makes sure that you are giving your child high quality calories, not empty calories from sugary foods. Babies are amazingly self-regulatory when it comes to their food intake. They eat when they're hungry and they stop when they're full.

Monitor your child's weight in consultation with your pediatrician, and only become concerned if you see wide aberrations in either direction.

Frequently Asked Questions

Glossary

A

areola — The darkened area of skin around the nipple.

C

calcium – An essential mineral for the formation of bones and teeth that is also instrumental in the proper clotting of blood, the transmission of nerve cells, and the contraction of muscles.

calorie – A calorie is a measurement for a unit of energy. It is used as a designation in rating the nutritional value of a given food.

colostrum — For the first few days after giving birth, a woman's breasts produce a thick, yellow liquid rich in calories and infection-fighting proteins. This colostrum is only made in limited quantities before the mature milk begins to flow, but it is important to the health of a newborn.

D

dietary fiber - Dietary fiber is derived from the cell walls of plants, and is an indigestible complex carbohydrate. There are two types, water-soluble and water-insoluble.

Glossary

E

engorgement — After a woman's body stops producing colostrum and mature milk begins to flow, her breasts will become very full, or "engorged". This condition can also happen if the breasts are producing more milk than is being consumed. Feeding the baby or using a breast pump relieves engorgement.

essential amino acids – The body does not have the ability to synthesize nine amino acids that are termed "essential." These include histidine, isoleucine, leucine, lysine, methionine, phenylalanine, theronine, tryptophan, and valine.

H

Hind milk — Toward the end of a feeding, the breast milk becomes higher in fat and is called "hind milk."

I

iron – Iron is an essential mineral that helps the blood to carry oxygen throughout the body. When there is a dietary deficiency of iron, anemia can be the result.

L

latching on — "Latching on" is the term used to describe the action of the baby properly taking the nipple and areola into the mouth for nursing.

Glossary

M

macronutrient – These are nutrients that form a major portion of a well-balanced diet, and are the major contributors to the creation of energy in the body. They include carbohydrates, fats, and protein.

milligram – A unit of measurement used in nutritional and supplemental descriptions. It equals one-thousandth of a gram (g).

N

nursing bra — Nursing bras are outfitted with flaps on the cups designed to be drawn aside to facilitate breastfeeding.

nursing pads – Small round pads designed to fit inside a bra for the purpose of absorbing leaking breast milk. The pads help to keep the woman's skin and clothing dry and free of infection and irritation.

P

potassium – An essential mineral necessary for the regulation of cardiac function, blood pressure, and nerve and muscle function.

protein – Proteins are a basic component of food and are built of amino acids. All of the body's enzymes and antibodies are proteins, as well as some hormones. Proteins transport oxygen and nutrients throughout the body and

Glossary

aid in the elimination of waste. They also build stronger muscles and tissues.

pumping — Pumping is the process of using an external pump, either manual or electric, to stimulate milk production in a nursing mother or to extract breast milk for storage and later use.

R

rooting reflex — A reflex triggered in children when something strokes their cheeks or lips causing them to begin searching for their mother's breast.

S

saturated fat - A fat or fatty acid that is typically solid at room temperature. Too much saturated fat in the diet leads to hardening of the arteries and coronary disease.

U

unsaturated fat – A fat or fatty acid that is typically a liquid at room temperature. Considered to be "good" fats.

V

Vitamin A – Among its other functions, Vitamin A is instrumental in the correct function of the eyes and the transmission of nerve signals to the retinas.

Glossary

Vitamin B1 – Vitamin B1 is needed by the body to break down carbohydrates, fat, and protein and is essential for proper nerve function.

Vitamin B2 – Vitamin B2 helps the body in processing amino acids and fats, and serves to help activate vitamin B6. It may also work as an antioxidant.

Vitamin B3 – Vitamin B3 is needed for cell respiration and for the release of the energy present in carbohydrates, fats, and proteins. It plays a role in supporting blood circulation, and is also necessary for healthy skin, nerve function, and the secretion of bile and digestive fluids in the stomach.

Vitamin B5 –Vitamin B5 works with the adrenal glands to transport and release energy from fats. It enables the synthesis of cholesterol and vitamin D.

Vitamin B6 – Vitamin B6 is crucial for immune system function and also aids in nerve function and the creation of healthy red blood cells.

Vitamin B9 – Often called folic acid, Vitamin B9 must be present for the replication and growth of cells. A lack of folic acid causes anemia.

Vitamin B12 – Vitamin B12 is necessary for normal nerve cell activity and the replication of DNA. Lack of Vitamin B12 causes fatigue.

Vitamin C – Vitamin C acts as an antioxidant and protects "good" cholesterol in the body from being damaged. It is

Glossary

necessary for the production of collagen, strengthens muscles and blood vessels, serves as an antihistamine, guards against cataracts, and strengthens immune function.

Vitamin D – Helps the body maintain proper levels of calcium in the blood and is necessary for strong bones and teeth. The body makes Vitamin D when it receives proper levels of sunshine, so in many areas, supplementation is required.

Vitamin E – The antioxidant Vitamin E protects cell membranes and reduces the risk of cardiovascular disease. It reduces levels of inflammation and encourages the growth of connective tissue.

Vitamin K – The body needs Vitamin K for blood coagulation and bone growth.

Index

acid reflux, 26, 36
amino acids, 72, 73
artificial colors, 56
asthma, 12
baby bottles, 41, 42, 43, 44, 45
bisphenol A (BPA), 37
blender, 51, 58, 62
blood, 30, 74, 75, 76, 83, 84
Bottles, 41, 42
botulism, 29, 56
brain, 26, 34, 37
burping, 47
cardiovascular disease, 26, 71, 74, 75
casein, 32
Celiac Disease, 55
childhood leukemia, 12
chloramine, 39, 40
Chlorine, 39
Choking, 53
colic, 36, 45
commercial baby food, 57
Concentrated liquid formulas, 37
constipation, 26
dental health, 26
diabetes (Type 1 and 2), 12
diarrhea, 31, 55, 83, 84
digestion, 26, 35
disinfection by-products, 39, 40
ear infections, 12, 26
endocrine system, 37
estrogen, 37
food processor, 58, 62
food safety, 68
fructose, 70, 71
gassiness, 55
glucose, 70
gluten, 58
gluten-free, 54
haloacetic acids, 40
hives, 55
ice cube trays, 64
immune system, 26, 28, 37
iron, 27, 31, 33, 50
iron-fortified formula, 33
irritability, 55
labored breathing, 55
lactation coach, 17
lactation specialists, 24
lacto-ovo vegetarian diet, 54
lactose, 70
latch, 19
latching on, 18
loose stools, 55
macronutrients, 70
maternity shop, 23
modified food starch, 58

Index

MSG, 58
municipal water systems, 39
nipples, 19, 42, 45
nursing bras, 23, 24
nursing pads, 22
omega-3 fatty acids, 26, 34
organic, 1, 39, 40, 58, 59
organics, 59, 60, 61, 62
ovarian cancers, 12
palmar grasp, 49
postpartum depression, 1, 12
powdered formulas, 36, 37
protein hydrolysate formulas, 35
pumps, 24, 25, 43
ready-to-use formulas, 37, 38
Ready-to-use formulas, 37
respiratory infections, 12
rice cereal, 50
runny nose, 55
sippy cups, 42
solid food, 49, 83
Soy-based formulas, 35
Stainless steel, 41
stomach viruses, 12
store breast milk, 21
sucrose, 70
Sudden Infant Death Syndrome (SIDS), 12
sugar, 28, 51, 58, 63, 70, 90
teeth, 76, 78, 89
Teething, 89
thrive, 15
tongue, 18, 19, 49, 55
toxic, 39, 41, 45
trans fats, 74, 76
trihalomethanes, 40
unsaturated fat, 74
vegan diet, 54
vegetarian, 54
Vitamin D, 27, 31, 77
volatile organic compounds, 40
vomiting, 26, 55
water supply, 37, 39
wet nurses, 29
whey proteins, 32

www.ingramcontent.com/pod-product-compliance
Lightning Source LLC
Chambersburg PA
CBHW060841050426
42453CB00008B/782